In memory of Ally and Logan

"Yesterday is a memory, tomorrow is a mystery and today is a gift and that is why we call it the present."

Author unknown

A View From Bed 15

A P a r e n t ' s P e r s p e c t i v e

The Story of an Organ Transplant for Zachary Johnson

12-19-2008

Thank you for following Zachary's plight. Thank you for your thoughts & prayers.
Brian & Deanna

by Brian K. Johnson

A View From Bed 15

Cover art and interior design by: Brian K. Johnson

ISBN 978-1-60145-681-6

www.booklocker.com

Printed in the United States of America

Table of Contents

Prologue

Having a child is an amazing experience. You go through the thrills of pregnancy, the act of delivery, and then the wonderful memories of childhood. This is the way that it is supposed to be. This is what parents look forward to. This is life as we know it.

However, sometimes life takes a turn in the wrong direction. Medical care is needed. Hospital visits are required; sometimes for extended days in a row. As parents we have to adapt our idea of what normal is and continue on with life. It is not an easy road to travel, but hopefully it is a temporary one. It is our wish that this will eventually lead back to the main highway of life...or rather that of a normal life.

But many times this road isn't temporary.

How do we as parents handle the day-to-day activities of a child in the hospital? How do we juggle the demands of house payments along with the needs of our children? Sometimes it is a tough balancing act to manage all while keeping our sense of sanity in check. It is a difficult position to say the least.

Just as there is no correct way of raising a child at home, there is no correct way of raising a child within a hospital. All of us strive to make the best decisions and sometimes we nail it on the head and other times we don't. After all, we are all human - we all march to a different drum.

This book encapsulates the story of a child who spent the first few years of his life within the walls of three hospitals. These writings portray a parent's perspective on the day-to-day visits and overnight stays in an ICU setting. Although our son, Zachary, occupied several bed locations over his hospital jaunts, the majority of his residency was at Bed 15 at Children's Hospital in Pittsburgh, PA. The following chapters narrate our struggles and fears in our child's life as well our sense of humor in a hospital setting.

Accompanying these following chapters are various journal entries from a web site devoted to Zachary. These blogs were originally intended to give brief updates and quick bits of information about Zachary's status. After a short amount of time these factoids on my son's health became a little more involved. Soon they were reflecting a parent's perspective on the idiosyncrasies of day-to-day hospital life.

There is no real explanation for the tone in the following blogs. Some depict the deep emotional feelings that I experienced in Zachary's daily medical roller coaster rides. Others relate to odd reflections or perceptions that Deanna and I had while hanging out in the various ICU locations.

After awhile the blogs morphed into my desire to tie together inexplicable links between childhood memories and present real life conditions. Sometimes these blogs were edited and rewritten before posting and other times I wrote off the cuff at 2am.

The orders of the blogs are chronological and placed after the most relative chapter. Hopefully, these placements add a sense of cohesion amongst the chapters and thus the book.

Our son's journey was a major inspiration for us. We gained an intense education in medical science, a tremendous following of a web-based audience, as well as the support of friends, family, and total strangers.

The following chapters and blogs are simply a collection of thoughts in a surreal and very scary situation all during a time when we were desperately trying to make sense of it all. It is our hope that you, the reader will find some common ground in these stories and perhaps share in some of the insights that Deanna and I experienced while watching over Zachary at Bed 15.

Chapter 1

The Beginning

Zachary Mason Johnson was born July 2, 2006 at the University Of Maryland Medical Center in Baltimore. He, along with twin brother Aidan, came into this world a few months earlier than we had planned – apparently setting the tone for what was going to be a very long childhood. A few hours prior to the birth I pulled into the hospital parking lot and enjoyed the warm and comforting feeling that the sun applied on my face.

"This is a good day to become a dad," I thought. With Deanna's overnight luggage in one hand and a cup of coffee in the other I was ready to take this monumental walk past the front entrance's rotating glass doors and into the maternity ward. These were steps that I wanted to savor for a few moments. All of our parenting plans came down to this. Parenthood was soon upon us.

But this story doesn't really start here. It actually started several years back in Seattle, Washington. The Pacific Northwest is a great place to live if you like nature, water ferries, and a big volcano looming over the horizon. Throughout our stay we took advantage of everything this area provided. We hiked. We kayaked. We slept in tents deep within Mt. Rainier National Park. Our lives were full of excitement in this city of rain, technology, and coffee.

Deanna and I had put off the "kid conversation" until she finished her studies and obtained her Master's degree in Physical Therapy from the University of Puget Sound in Tacoma, Washington. During this time I worked as a database developer for a national real estate company up the road in the nearby community of SeaTac. It's not that we didn't want children. It's just that they didn't factor into our lives at this point in time. After

Deanna's graduation we sort of threw caution to the wind and embarked on a two month backpacking trip around Europe.

Prior to our trip we had sold our house in Seattle and put all of our belongings in a 10x10 foot storage bin. Nothing like knowing that your whole life can be stored away in a small cubical protected from the evils of the world by a $4 padlock. Still, the world was ours for the taking...provided that the price was low enough.

Now it is important to note that we are adults of...shall I say...a frugal nature? Perhaps it is our modest Midwest raising or the fact that our careers took us along a lower paying route. Either way, we didn't have a ton of money to spend when hiking around some of Europe's most beautiful cities. We chose picnics instead of pricy restaurants, we opted to stay in hostels instead of hotels, and when a cheap hostel wasn't available, we actually spent the night in a barn. Okay, so that only happened once but hopefully this shows some insight into our budget-minded spending habits.

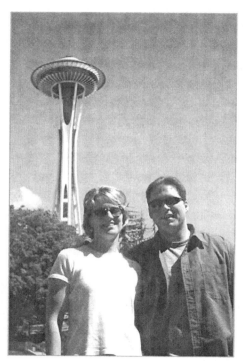

Deanna & Brian in Seattle

Our story actually gains some momentum on the final leg of our backpacking trip. At this time we found ourselves smack dab in the middle of Paris, France. It was a very beautiful day as we sat in the park overlooking the Eiffel Tower. With a picnic lunch spread out before us we confessed that our lives were pretty good. We were newly married, young, and had no responsibilities.

It was at that moment that everything seemed clear. The life that we led was a prelude to the life that we would lead. Our knowledge and experience were stepping-stones to a future of prosperity and happiness. Everything was falling in line. Life was becoming simpler. It was time to take the next step in our relationship. The obvious was staring us in the face.

Lose the birth control.

And thus our destiny was set in motion.

That defining moment was July 2, 2001 and from that point on nothing had gone according to plan. Conception never occurred and pregnancy never developed. Throughout this ordeal we adopted a nomadic approach to living and moved several times resembling some sort of bizarre witness relocation episode. To be fair, most of the moves were job related which took us from Seattle to Cleveland to San Francisco back to Seattle and finally to Maryland. But throughout most of this endeavor the pregnancy thing never took. Maybe it was bad timing on the ovulation front. Maybe my underwear was too tight. Maybe we just weren't doing it right. Who knows?

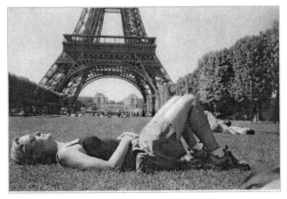
Deanna in Eiffel Park, Paris

Sometime in Seattle (the second time around that is) we decided to pry open the checkbook and invest in Invitro Fertilization (IVF). Consider this approach a combination of nature, test tubes, Petri dishes and a squadron of trained medical personnel. It seems the last resort and dare I say the most expensive. Not exactly the preferred path of frugal people. But after a handful of appointments and tests it all came down to a positive blood test. Deanna was pregnant...with twins.

We logged a lot of miles from that day in Paris to delivery day in Baltimore. In the end it took us exactly five years to the day, thousands of dollars of our own money and the help of IVF doctors to make our joys of parenthood a reality. Not exactly the time frame that we were looking for but dwelling on the past was never our style.

We have always enjoyed the proximity of living near water and thus it wasn't any surprise that we sought out coastal Maryland as an ideal location for our new lives. Now we live in Severna Park, Maryland - a small bedroom community located just upstream from the Chesapeake Bay. It is a beautiful place to live and very close to historic Annapolis. As the pregnancy progressed we kind of developed this fantasy of hanging out in an Annapolis coffee shop on a Sunday morning with our dog and twin boys. Just like on the cover of an LL Bean catalog.

Chapter 2

The Twins Enter This World

On July 1, 2006. Deanna and I were getting all of our ducks in a row for the birth of the twins. We had already done the Lamaze classes. We had scoped out the best route to the hospital – with and without traffic. We even had plans for painting the nursery an appropriate baby boy blue color on the very next day. We had the paint, the drop cloth, and all of the brushes sitting inside the hallway. If anything, we were on the verge of over planning. No problem, since the twins' expected due date was August 29, 2006 we had a few more months to get it all done.

At around midnight Deanna woke me up to inform me that her water had broken. It took a few seconds for my sleep barrier to break down and this news to grab a foothold in my consciousness. Once my brain grasped the importance of the situation I realized that I had to do something. Fatherhood instincts kicked in gear! Eons of paternal evolution were now taking over. I was a pawn to my ancestral DNA. Immediately I jumped out of bed and...stood there. I had absolutely no idea of what to do.

We may have planned for a lot of stuff along this pregnancy route but one thing was for certain; we didn't plan on this. Panic, gibberish and walking in circles quickly morphed into getting the bags packed, getting the car warmed up, and making sure that Deanna was in the passenger seat. Looking back, I've come to the conclusion that including Deanna in my trip to the hospital was very important to a successful delivery.

The trip to the hospital proved to be the starting point to a series of odd events. Our master plan was to have the twins delivered at Greater Baltimore Medical Center. Once there Deanna was quickly registered and put in a somewhat dark and quiet room to await the inevitable birth. The electronic wires were connected to my wife's belly for the sole purpose of monitoring the twin's vital signs. The only noises we heard were the amplified sounds of the babies' heartbeats, which were sounding eerily similar to the sound effects from *A Space Odyssey*.

So here we were. Just the two of us in a dark nurturing room passing the time until we officially became parents. Again, life took a different path. Unfortunately a nurse (whom I assuming drew the short straw from her coworkers) won the job of telling my pregnant wife that she couldn't stay and would have to leave. As it turns out, the hospital did not have any open beds for our sons. To make matters worse, the nursing staff was having difficulty finding a hospital to accept us. It seems as if Baltimore was having a mini baby boom that night. All the delivery rooms in the area were full. Now we know how Mary and Joseph felt.

Eventually we got a verbal acceptance from the University of Maryland Medical Center (UMMC) and before I knew it, three official looking medical people were wheeling Deanna out of the room and down the hallway to an awaiting ambulance. Of course, there was no room in the ambulance for me. After all, I'm just the father of the soon to be delivered twin boys. Somewhere in the baby manual it must state that dad's wants and desires are meaningless. It is a cruel fact of life. I had best be getting used to it.

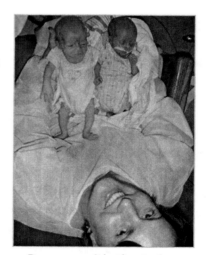

Deanna with the twins

Time to skip back to the part about me enjoying the sun on my face. After entering the UMMC hospital I found my way up to some sort of prep room for expecting mothers. "I'm not in Kansas anymore", I mumbled. This area resembled a meteorologist headquarters during a hurricane. There were lots of people hurrying around in fast motion and lots of conversations in a language that I didn't quite understand. The medical folks were jockeying around my wife doing this, doing that. Not a lot of empty areas for a clueless father-to-be to hang out. I surveyed the room and spied a small island of usable space in the corner and made a bee line for that space.

Feeling useless and totally out of my element I tried my best to resemble the star quarterback during the fourth quarter rally. I talked to Deanna in a calm reassuring manner but she was on a totally different plane and not really listening to me at all. The doctor was in charge here and I quickly realized that I'm not anywhere near quarterback status but more like the team mascot.

In a rare moment, the doctor pulls me aside and tells me that it would be best to delay my wife's delivery - something about the babies' continuing development or something of this nature. It is probably important to note that everything is happening really fast and I'm still proud of the fact that I actually found this hospital. After all, the ambulance driver from the first hospital didn't really make it easy for me. He gave me a bad map to UMMC and said "see you there".

So here I am listening to the doctor as he talks to me about something important. I wasn't sure if he wanted a reply from me or for me just to be quiet. During a pause in his dialogue I commented that it would be cool to tell my friends that the twins were born on the Fourth of July. Perhaps he could delay the birth by a few more days. The look that he gave me had the word moron written all over it. Okay, so I missed his point completely ...whatever it was. I was nervous and tried the humorous approach. In hindsight, I should have chosen the quiet route. To be honest, even to this day I still think that having my boys born on the Fourth of July would have been pretty cool.

In the end, Aidan and Zachary were born that afternoon. During the delivery I sat by Deanna's side in some special daddy chair and was told not to move. For the most part, I listened to Dr. Do-As-I-Say-Or-Else and watched both boys enter the world in awe. Aidan (3lb, 2oz) was born first. Zachary (2lb, 10oz) popped out a few minutes later. With both babies' bundled in a cotton blanket I had the opportunity to hold them briefly. It's a moment that I'll always cherish. One thing that stands out though is with Zachary. While holding my second born I remember that he opened his left eye and surveyed Dad for a few seconds. An apparent wink as it were. That was a very cool moment.

So Deanna and I have now gained membership into the exclusive Parent's Club of America. We were happy and excited to the power of 10. To celebrate we called everyone we could think of and actually reached a few of our friends. All I can say is good thing for voicemail. Like I thought earlier that morning in the parking lot, it was a good day to be a dad... even though this day came seven weeks earlier than expected; it was a good day nevertheless.

Chapter 3

Aidan Comes Home

About three weeks after the twin's birth, Deanna and I were able to bring Aidan home. Although Zachary still needed a little more time to get stronger we felt that this was a "one baby at a time" evolution process. When we worked out the kinks with one kid then, good timing permitted, then we would be ready to bring home another. Perhaps life was turning out peachy keen after all – especially for me. After all Aidan was a cute baby who slept a lot and really didn't make much noise. However, my Father Knows Best scenario of watching child rearing from afar came crashing down on me.

Apparently Aidan required the routine midnight feedings and diaper changing. Since Mother Nature had not instilled me with the necessary plumbing I naturally assumed that it would be Deanna who would be getting out of bed every two hours. My job was to support Deanna (in spirit only of course) from the confines of a warm and comfortable bed. Why should I have to get up? After all,

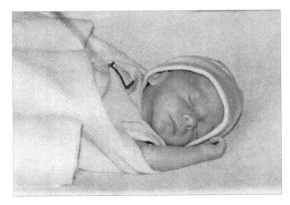

Aidan at home napping

this duty was obviously tailored for the female of the species. At least that was my thought.

I guess I thought wrong.

There was a major flaw in my thought process. This was not my grand dad's generation or for that matter my dad's. Times had changed and ingenuity had somehow caught up with the present. Someone, somewhere long ago had invented something called "the Bottle". It was a strategic device intended to make life easier for mothers and hell for the fathers. I was informed that I was just as qualified to get up and feed Aidan while Deanna applied the medieval device commonly referred to as a breast pump on her overflowing breasts. It didn't look comfortable and certainly wasn't enjoyable. I quickly realized that this was one battle that I would never win. So up every two hours became the new plan for myself.

Our sleep schedules would never be the same.

Since we were getting the hang of Aidan's requirements and a sleep deprived ability to work at our jobs we started to get a little anxious about bringing Zachary home. After all, we had the nursery set up with not one, but two cribs. Two of everything actually - two car seats, two monogrammed bath towels and two matching blue baby blankets. But life decided to throw us a curve; Zachary would be staying away from home a little while longer.

Chapter 4

Zachary's Introduction To Surgery

About three weeks into Zachary's NICU stay we knew something wasn't right. His belly was getting somewhat swollen which meant that his feeds were not traveling south to his diaper. In other words, something was plugging up his pipes. The doctors were watching him very carefully and keeping us up to date on the situation. Even though they explained the whole thing in very easy to follow terms, we had no idea just what was fixable and what wasn't.

Personally, I asked as many questions as I could think of. Some of the questions were relevant to the situation but most were probably way out in left field and had absolutely no connection to Zachary's

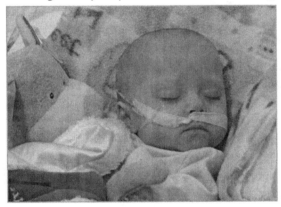

Zachary after his 1st surgery

intestinal tract. The thing is that I had no idea what was relevant or what wasn't. It was like I was thrown into the deep end of the pool and expected to find my way back to the shallow end.

Through it all, I didn't care if I came across as a highly trained medical student or an uneducated tree trimmer (no offense to those in the arbor business). I was on a fact-finding mission. Gastrointestinal science was not my college minor so I was desperately trying to play catch up. The way I figured it, too much information was not necessarily a bad thing. Connecting the medical dots was now my highest priority and I was going to ask as many questions as it took to figure this out. But the crash course in Zachary's medical dilemma wouldn't be accomplished in one day. Learning my fair share of pediatric gastrointestinal knowledge would have to wait a little while longer.

The next day, I got a call on my work phone that Zachary's belly had gotten worse and that his life was now in jeopardy. The time for waiting it out was now over. Surgery was needed right away. The doctor requested me to come to the NICU immediately and sign a consent form. My office was ten minutes away from the hospital and that day I made it over there in five. Deanna arrived a few minutes after me and like myself tried to concentrate on the essential facts and make sense of this rapidly changing scenario.

The surgeon who had been following the situation over the past few days told us in a calm manner that Zachary had something called Necrotizing Enterocolitis or NEC. This is a gastrointestinal disease that kills the tissue in and around the bowel wall. Without healthy tissue the food cannot be absorbed or, more importantly, cannot pass through - hence the blockage. This is not a common disease in the world of pediatrics but it shows up enough to have some

> *necrotizing* means the death of tissue,
> *entero* refers to the small intestine,
> *col* refers to the colon,
> *itis* means inflammation.

statistics behind it. NEC affects mostly premature infants - 1 in every 2000 on average.

As the surgeon continued his dialogue my mind couldn't help but drift off to my son laying innocently in his climate-controlled isolette. He looked so peaceful and comfortable. How could the surgeon possible want to interrupt this baby's nap with a scalpel? Was this really happening? As I toggled my attention between his statements and my son's presence I realized that other medical type people started entering the room. The anesthesiologist was beginning to gather his own information about Zac in order to create the appropriate sedation for surgery. Various Operating Room techs were beginning to mull around the room in anticipation of wheeling Zachary away.

"Do you have any questions?" the surgeon asked. As the reality of the situation came racing up close and personal I glanced over at Deanna in hope that she was following the conversation much better than I was. Thankfully she asked a few questions which helped me to regroup and focus on the matter at hand. The surgeon's answers helped a little but failed to answer the most important question. Why did Zachary get this? Well, no one knew that answer. It was just plain bad luck commingled with the fact that he was a preemie and a hundred other non-definable reasons.

The where's, why's and how's really weren't important at this stage. Zachary needed to be fixed and surgery was the last option. We signed the consent form and watched our son get wheeled away by total strangers in blue surgical scrubs. It was at that moment that our lives took a hard right turn into the unknown. Hearing the diagnosis was just the beginning. We would have several days to understand this disease - and many months to deal with it. It was going to become a long and mentally exhausting experience. The extent of which would not be known for well over two years.

Chapter 5

The Surgical Waiting Room

T he University of Maryland Medical Center has one of the nicer places to pass time than any other hospital that I have seen. It is a balcony of sorts with trees and surprisingly very comfortable chairs, couches and benches. In fact, if this balcony were located anywhere else it would make an ideal setting for a prom or a great spot for an Olive Garden. This waiting area has plenty of today's newspapers strewn about – probably by other surgery related relatives in the same position as Deanna and myself. You can only read so many articles about the Iraq War, the governor or the mayor before you crave a magazine by Martha Stewart or if desperate enough - Teen Beat.

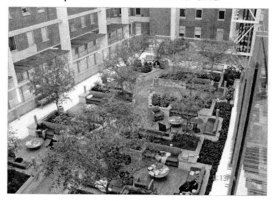

UMMC waiting room

After a few hours of waiting around with no additional information you naturally start to get a little nervous. You start to wonder just how things are going and contemplate sticking your head into the Operating Room door just to get a little information. Thankfully, the OR liaison told us that if we had questions to consult with the waiting room personnel located at the front of the area. "Just have her call the OR for updates", she said. Since I have never been in an Operating Room during an operation I really had no preconception on how this worked. Was it the doctor's duty to pick up the phone for the update? Was there a nurse whose sole job was to simply answer the phone? Perhaps a Bluetooth head set on the surgeon's assistant for such an occasion. Perhaps this was more of a Bat Phone setup where the waiting room attendant simply picked up her phone (bypassing Commissioner Gordon in the process) and automatically made the phone ring in the Operating Room.

After all of this heavy and intense mental pondering I decided to just go up and ask. Let the powers at large handle all of the complicated communication engineering feats. As I stood by with my half empty cold cup of coffee I watched the waiting room attendant call the operating room with a simple four number code and heard the following: "I'm calling about Zachary Johnson's status"..."Yes"..."Okay"..."Sure"..."Uh-huh"..."Uh-huh"..."How long?"..."Really?"..."I'll tell him. Thank you".

She then hangs up the phone, turns to me and says, "He's fine". "What? That's it?" I asked. "Cause it sounded like they said a lot more than that". "Nope", He's fine," she mumbled. Apparently parents are on a medical need-to-know basis when it comes to information on your child.

Not to be deterred, I then rattled off several key questions relating to Zachary's medical condition and drug related issues. Shortly after I began this rapid fire of questions I realized that this lady had as much interest in my affairs as a vegetarian at a butcher's shop. She nodded politely and gave me the same answer: "Your son is doing fine". Not quite the data retrieving adventure that I had hoped. It was a long walk back to the bench where Deanna was sitting. "He's fine" I said with the confidence only an award winning actor could portray.

A few hours (and several hundred feet of pacing) later the surgeon emerged from the double doors near the waiting room. He approached with his surgical scrubs still in place. "All went well", he immediately stated. Whew! Time to take a good deep breath and let the lungs continue their course of action. The surgeon went on to describe how he had to cut away several centimeters of bowel that had essentially been killed off by the disease. Of course, I am not a Metrics kinda guy and was diverting valuable brain processing power trying to convert his measurement into inches. Then it dawned on me that I really had no idea just how many inches of bowel a baby has in his belly anyway.

At this time the conversion really didn't matter. The surgery was done. Zachary was doing fine and life would resume in a normal fashion a few months later than expected.

Chapter 6

Adjusting to Maryland

E ven though Zachary was still in the hospital recovering from his first of many surgeries we still had to keep some semblance of a normal life. Of course, "normal" is such a misunderstood word these days. Ask five people to describe the word "normal" and you will most likely receive five different definitions. But no matter what definition you choose, one thing is for certain: the bills still needed to be paid. The bank expected a check every month for the house payment. Food had to be put on the table and the electric company didn't take I.O.U.'s. In short, we needed jobs to keep going.

Now, it is not like we are irresponsible people. We did have some sort of a plan of attack here. A few months before we sold our house in Seattle, Deanna had interviewed and accepted a position as a part-time Pediatric Physical Therapist at a hospital just north of Baltimore. Somehow during the interviewing process she was told that she would receive full time benefits for her part time position. It was a pretty sweet deal actually. Quite the negotiator is my wife.

During this two month period Deanna, not only being pregnant with twins, found and bought our house in Severna Park as well as a vehicle tailored to a couple with two kids and a dog. With this in mind I figured that I had best get business wrapped up in Seattle and hightail it to Maryland before she spent any more of our money. After the birth of the twins, she received her standard twelve-week maternity leave as well as a tremendous amount of support from her coworkers. She had carried the twins, gave birth to the twins and was now caring for Aidan and making the daily trip to visit with Zachary. She had done her part and more.

Prior to the twins' birth I had obtained a one-year database contract gig with a local utility company. The money was decent, the type of work was right up my alley, and the short commute time was something I could live with. I figured that this was a good job in the interim to make ends meet until our whirlwind tour of life settled down a little. You know, looking back we realized that life never did settle down. Not even a little.

Coming off of a few contracting gigs at Seattle based Microsoft I was used to the intense pressure of getting the job done yesterday. When you work for someone who works for someone who works for the richest man in the world you tend to accelerate your pace to superhuman speed. The trick, of course, is to drink lots and lots of Seattle based Starbucks coffee. Hmm, now that I think of it I'm sure that the two corporate powers had this in mind all along. Diabolical! Anyway, back to my new gig, it didn't take me long to get the hang of what my new boss wanted. Within a month or so I had improved their departmental number crunching process with a few extra lines of computer code. In fact, I turned an 8-hour day into a 4-hour day.

You see, we database developers, or chip heads as we are often referred to, are essentially a lazy bunch. We would rather have a computer do all of the work as opposed to actually doing anything that resembles work. So in order to avoid work the second time around we spent lots of time writing code the first time around. I could explain this better but I would need various charts and graphs to make my point. Basically, we add as many lines of code as needed to accomplish the task at hand. The end result is a "click here" button and the sight of the computer guy walking away to the coffee stand.

Shortly after the new and improved database was rolled off of the caffeine assembly line the twins were born - and shortly after that was the news of Zachary's disease. Even though the utility company's management was sympathetic with my situation they still expected me to be there on time and get my work done. To be honest, getting the job done really wasn't the issue. Since my workload was now reduced four hours a day the biggest challenge was to look busy the other four hours.

With extra time on my hands, Aidan at home and Zachary in the NICU (Neonatal Intensive Care Unit) I couldn't just sit on my hands and wait for my paycheck. Add to this the fact that my desk had no windows to look through; I was getting bored with my job. It was time for a change. So I took on a few more internal assignments and negotiated the use of a company laptop and the ability to work offsite. The result was that my conscious was clear regarding an 8-hour a day paycheck and I got to hang out with Zachary while he vacationed at Club NICU. So the corporate juggling act commonly referred to as "work-life-balance" was now in full swing.

Chapter 7

W e b   B a s e d   S u p p o r t

A t this time, it became apparent that there were a large amount of family and friends who were following Zachary's plight. In the beginning it was reasonable to pass this information along with phone calls, but with the list of interested people kept growing. Add to this the fact that many of these folks were on the west coast (note the 3 hour time difference) it soon became very time consuming and frankly our cell phone minutes were about to run out. This, of course, was good for our cell phone carrier, but bad for our bank balance.

So we needed a better form of communication. Sending out emails with multiple addresses seemed to be the wise approach. However, some of our addresses were outdated and it took too much energy to track down which Yahoo! account was the most recent. Since modern technology didn't really remind us to update our electronic Rolodex, the email approach proved to be more of an irritant. So the search for a better mousetrap was once again under way.

It was Deanna's idea to convey Zachary's progress through the use of various Internet sites. She found a domain site located at Carepage.com (and eventually later at COTA.com), which enabled us to post journals, photos, as well as the ability for others to post supporting comments or statements of hope. Basically, these web sites were a conduit between us and anyone who wanted to follow Zachary's progress.

These sites were ideal as we were able to post his condition, his medications, and our opinions on how the nurses and/or doctors interacted with our NICU son. In fact, it worked so well that I started to provide more of our insights and nuances into everyday hospital occurrences as it related to a parent of a child in the hospital. As we quickly learned, when one visits the hospital on a daily basis there can be a lot of insights. The amount of material that I could write about appeared limitless.

Of course, my style of writing was more on a therapeutic level than anything else. It quickly became my way of dealing with some very serious issues surrounding the health of my son. Sometimes the journal entries are direct and void of humorous insights while others tended to stray away from Zachary's medical mumbo-jumbo and focus on hospital pet peeves. Whatever the approach, the blogs are intended to share parental viewpoints of a hospital setting.

In the process, however, the web sites doubled as a communication tool between Zachary's ICU status and our list of family and friends. As time went on, the list of family and friends grew to include acquaintances. Then the list grew to include people we didn't know. According to the number of hits on Zachary's web site it was apparent that there are a lot of people we don't know.

Word of mouth got this ball rolling initially. Soon, articles by the Severna Park paper spread to the Annapolis News and then to Fox News and the ball just kept rolling. Perhaps people were visiting the site for inspiration. Perhaps they could relate to our "fish out of water" experiences within the hospital. Either way the list of people following Zachary's progress was growing every day.

Chapter 8

The Endless Wait

A few months had gone by since Zachary's surgery. His bowel was healing quite nicely and the swelling, due to the operation, had subsided. His sedation was decreased on a daily basis and thus he was awake more and more. In general terms, he was getting better. The doctors had even reintroduced feeds back into his belly through the use of an NG tube.

For those of you who haven't watched any NG episodes on the Medical Channel, let me bring you up to date. An NG tube, or Nasal Gastrointestinal tube is a small diameter sized flexible plastic tube that is inserted through the nose of the patient all the way down to the stomach. It is the best way to feed a patient who, like Zachary, hasn't mastered the intricacies of bottle-feeding. It is also the preferred way as the nurse can monitor and track the amount of feed volume that Zachary is actually receiving. Inserting the tube was probably irritating for Zachary, but once in, he barely noticed it. In reality, it is probably more painful for the parents to watch than anything else.

A basic indicator on how the bowel's plumbing was working was measured by just how much of the liquid feed Zachary could tolerate. Like most post operations, you had to progress slowly. At first the feeds were a trickle actually – 5 ml per hour. Then if all looked good that amount was increased to 10 ml/hr and so on and so on. Ultimately the goal was to reach 60 ml/hr. According to my calculations, this figure looked attainable within a week or so.

The NEC disease was certainly a serious issue and really set Zachary's health back several months. But by the looks of everything it appeared to have been beaten. Zachary was getting fed more every day. His weight was increasing and we were able to pick him up without coordinating permission from the nurse, the doctor, and any hospital administrators. We were back on track to getting Zachary all healed up and discharged from the hospital.

Once again, life didn't go according to plan. We watched Labor Day (Sep 4, 2006) pass with Zachary in the NICU. Same went for Halloween (Oct 31, 2006) and Veteran's Day (Nov 11, 2006). Apparently my calculations for a discharge date were missing a few unknown variables. Progress in this area was small and at times stagnant.

In the meantime, we were becoming familiar with everything connected with hospitals. We knew exactly when the Starbucks kiosk opened or the price of the chocolate chip cookies at The Great Cookie hut. Even the rotating weekly specials at the hospital café were becoming memorized. Not to mention the names of the nurses, their spouses or where they went to college.

Then on November 16, 2006 all of the time consuming progress was wiped away. Zachary's NEC had returned and he was rushed into emergency surgery. Once again we spent time on the tree lined waiting area. Once again we waited for the surgeon to come out and tell us that everything went well. And once again, Zachary will be without even more of his intestines.

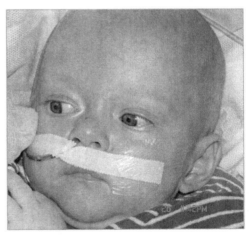

Things couldn't possibly get any worse. But like a

Zachary with NG tube

very bad dream it did. Three days later it was apparent that the intestinal tissues were not doing well. Once again the surgical team was summoned and once again operated on this tough little baby. The surgeon told us that they found about 40 centimeters (roughly

16 inches) of bad intestine and cut it away. At this point Zachary was down to about half of his original bowel length.

After several hours of unsuccessfully trying to make sense of it all, Deanna and I returned to the crib side and resumed our parental duties of being there for Zachary. He was now very swollen and connected to several IV's pumping appropriate medicines into his body for the sake of recovery. It will be several weeks before we could hold him again. In the meantime we sat by his crib and stared at him, held his hand, and hoped for the best.

Our once firm plans of having the twins home together for the holidays soon evaporated. We now watched Thanksgiving Day (Nov 23, 2006) pass with Zachary in the NICU. The same went for Christmas (Dec 25, 2006) and New Years Day (Jan 1, 2007).

Chapter 9

Attempt at Normalcy

Throughout it all we continued to raise Aidan like any normal child. He went on stroller rides around the neighborhood, had play dates, and interacted with the grand parents on a regular basis. We were especially appreciative of the NICU staff for allowing Aidan to visit Zachary as often as possible as this allowed for some form of bonding session with his twin. Many times, we had both boys on a mat on the floor playing with toys getting to know each other. Aidan was okay staying in one place for a short amount of time while Zachary, although tethered to the crib with various tubes and lines, was content to hang out with big brother. It wasn't *Leave it to Beaver*, but it worked for us.

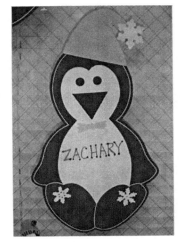

Zachary's plaque at NICU

This was now our life – or rather our adaptation of life. Of course, the more time we spent at the NICU, the more comfortable we became. We now entered the room like it was our own dormitory. We chatted with the nurses like they were our roommates. With the exception of a few of the doctors, we were pretty much on a first name basis. The "No Beverages in the NICU" rule didn't seem to apply to me anymore (although I still continued to hide it from view). Outside of our home, we spent more time here than anywhere else.

But as time consuming as the NICU was, we still managed to give quality time to Aidan. It was a balancing act for sure, but not one that required a whole lot of thought. Deanna and I had developed a routine that allowed for at least one parent to be with Aidan during the day and after the work hours we traded off to be with Zachary. During the weekends, we had even more flexibility for the twins.

Of course, there was some degree of give and take here as there are only so many hours in a day. For instance, the grass got mowed only when small caribou started grazing on our lawns. Automobile maintenance occurred when the dashboard's red light emerged and the laundry was done whenever time permitted. We learned not to stress over small stuff, but to deal with life in a much different perspective. There was certainly a new order of priorities we were now facing. It seemed so obvious now. How did we miss this throughout the beginning of our lives? Did anyone else know about this?

Of course, it would be a crime to suggest that we did this alone. At this point, word got out among the neighbors about the new couple with the twins, the border collie, the disease and the surgeries. Neighbors, those we knew and those we didn't, dropped off meals for our consumption. It seemed that many of these folks had a friend or relative who, at some point in time, had been in the hospital and could thus relate to our new lifestyle. These were incredible gestures of kindness and generosity that we never expected.

Our neighborhood of Severna Park, MD is called Cape Arthur. It is named this due to the location of the houses and the beach area – long named after the developer Arthur Giddings. The neighborhood is off the beaten path of the shopping areas and main drag of Severna Park. There are no sidewalks, no lights or shortcuts from one area of town to another. Only a few speed bumps to coax a would be NASCAR soccer mom to slow the minivan down a little. So it goes without saying that our neck of the woods is a slow paced alcove of homes with a lower than average turnover of residents.

During our strolls with Aidan, we routinely came across neighbors who were very much aware of Zachary's plight and desire to know more. The "Zac Grapevine" as I like to call it usually kept most of the neighbors up to speed on what seemed to be a daily occurrence. Still, the simple question about Zachary's condition, when asked, was always very much appreciated.

Both sets of grandparents drove from their Ohio homes to help us out. Actually, it really didn't take much prodding to get them to visit. Grandparents and grandchildren seem to go hand in hand – regardless of distance. Both Deanna's and my parents were incredible during this lengthy ordeal. They were always there when we needed them. No questions asked.

No matter the perspective, life was far from normal. However, in spite of it all we were starting to develop a daily routine that kept our sanity in check.

Chapter 10

The Omegaven Factor

A round November 2006, Zachary was taking small amounts of feed from a bottle. It was a token amount of fluid intended to get him used to bigger things down the road like Oreos and peanut butter sandwiches. But this low intake of feed wasn't nearly enough to keep him going. Throughout it all, he needed supplemental nutrition and lots of it. But how do you give a child with bad plumbing enough food to survive?

Enter the world of TPN & lipids.

- TPN (Total Parental Nutrition) is a concoction of various nutrients like salts, sugars, proteins, and various vitamins all rolled up into a liquid resembling Gatorade.
- Lipids are essentially a fatty composite in liquid form that has the general look and texture of whole milk.

These two forms of IV food don't store too well in the same container and thus are most efficient if kept separate. When needed they are injected into the body through separate lines. Sorta like your basic food and drink. Don't understand?

Let me try this analogy: Visualize a fine Sunday morning breakfast at Denny's consisting of toast, eggs, hash browns, and milk. The toast, eggs, and hash browns represent the mix of ingredients in TPN. The milk represents the lipids. Would you want to mix your toast, eggs, and hash browns with your milk in say, a large mixing bowl and eat with a spoon? I think not. Combined, these ingredients don't work. Taken separately though, the meal becomes a hit. This is probably why the Grand Slam breakfast meal has made this chain a fortune.

Let us return back to the medical field. The TPN is pumped into the patient's body separately with the lipids via an opening like an IV line, or in Zachary's case, a more semi-permanent central line. Basically, it is a way of feeding people who cannot eat by mouth. In the short term, this dynamic duo of TPN & lipids is a great way of providing nutrients to just about anyone. However this liquid magic pill has a dark side – it is very hard on the liver. In long-term patients, the use generally causes some rather horrific side effects...like liver failure. So the next question is how do you feed a child with TPN/lipids without hurting the liver?

Enter the World Wide Web. For me, the internet is a great resource for getting up to date scores on my favorite college football games. All I have to do is type in ESPN on my web browser and voila! Up pops several links to satisfy all of the sports craving needs that my little heart possesses. Whoever set this up was a genius. The invention of the Internet has certainly saved me from flipping on every cable channel in hope of catching the sports summary. Apparently you can use the Internet for other forms of data too. Who knew how long this was going on?

One day Deanna rolled up her sleeves and did some investigating on her own. Bypassing ESPN she discovered that there was a product currently being used by patients on TPN/lipids in institutions such as Children's Hospital in Boston that wasn't harmful on the liver. This amazing product was called Omegaven.

Omegaven is a substitution for the lipids compound used in conjunction with TPN. Where lipids are made from a fatty soybean based component, Omegaven uses an Omega 3 fatty fish oil component. Someone somewhere must have deduced that since fish don't get liver disease then they must hold the key to our liver dilemma – or at least that is my theory. From what we were able to read, Omegaven helped slow down, stop or even reverse the trend of the liver failure among these patients. Admittedly it is still in some sort of study phase but the initial results were very impressive.

Now before anyone decides to mortgage their home on Omegaven stock let me temper this urge by stating that this drug is still in the experimental stages. Nothing has been 100% proven yet but my biased gut feels that the jury may be leaning towards granting some sort of Nobel Prize for fishy based human IV food.

So Deanna contacted everyone from the staff at the Boston hospital where this Internet article spoke about to parents who have their child on Omegaven. Soon emails were arriving from other parents whose children were on the drug in the past to those who are still actively receiving the drug. Most everyone that we spoke with praised this product enormously. With Zachary's liver starting to show signs of deterioration, could Omegaven be his wonder drug?

Since no one could say with any certainly just how long Zachary's liver would last with the current TPN/lipid setup, we decided to move forward with the addition of Omegaven. Of course this wasn't as easy as just signing on the dotted line. For starters, let me once again state that this drug was EXPERIMENTAL. In the medical field the word "experimental" has all of the red flags as lead based paint.

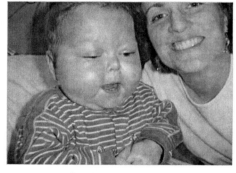

Zachary with Deanna

Another hurdle is the fact that no one at the University of Maryland Medical Center was currently on Omegaven. So we would have to be the path makers in getting this drug approved by the hospital's powers at large. And of course since Omegaven is <say it with me out loud> "Experimental", then it is not covered by insurance. So the big question for the UMMS accounting department was obvious. Who was going to pay for this? At approximately $100/day, this was beyond the financial means of Deanna and myself.

Shortly after bringing up the Omegaven issue with hospital officials, Deanna and I were given the strong impressions that if we wanted Zachary to receive Omegaven then he would have to go to Boston Children's. So within a few weeks Deanna and I had looked and narrowed out our choices of housing in the Boston area (and we thought that the Annapolis area was expensive). We worked out the logistics of her living in Boston and myself staying in Baltimore and continuing with my job. We even received approval from our insurance company to finance Zachary's medical flight to Boston.

But the trip to Bean Town was not in the cards. I would say that the helicopter was just about to get fueled up when UMMS made their decision. The use of Omegaven was approved. We were staying in Maryland.

Of course, it helps that we had some allies in this cause. One of the pediatric associate professors, who incidentally was one of the original members of the Zachary Johnson Fan Club, was totally on our side. Although the decision-making meeting was behind locked doors and subject to the same secrecy of the Patriot Act, we suspect that it was her who pushed for the acceptance or Omegaven.

Well, there were a lot of behind the scenes negotiations going on but let me sum it up via the bullet point method:

- Parents want Omegaven
- UMMS denies use of Omegaven
- Parents move forward and make arrangements to move Zachary to Boston hospital where he will receive Omegaven.
- Just a theory here, but I suspect that UMMS used basic math in determining how much money a pediatric patient brings into the income side of the budget vs. how much Omegaven costs on the expense side of the budget.
- UMMS reevaluates decision
- UMMS grants use and absorbs financial cost of Omegaven

The decision was made on January 11, 2007 – my birthday. I couldn't have been happier.

Chapter 11

The Liver, Workhorse of the Body

The liver is a marvel of engineering. It does so much for the human body and receives probably the least amount of coverage. Take in comparison the heart. Now heart transplants get much more publicity among newspapers and television programs. In fact, there are whole hospital wings devoted just for the transplant of such an organ. The simple fact is that the heart is a pump - pure and simple. Don't get me wrong – it is a very valuable pump and the plumbing and wiring of this organ is all very complex. But it has just one function: to move high volumes of blood.

The lungs too receive a lot of coverage and in all fairness tend to do a tad more work than the heart. Essentially the lungs' job is to inflate and deflate all while adding oxygen to the blood and taking carbon dioxide out. Consider it the Shop Vac of the human body.

The liver on the other hand does a whole lot more than a few functions. First of all, it is the largest gland in the body and is the only one that has the ability to regenerate itself. It is estimated that the liver has over 500 functions. It partners up with the stomach to help in the digestion of food. It makes bile, which is instrumental in the breakdown of fats. It filters toxins like ammonia and bilirubin. The liver makes chemicals, fights infections and kicks poisons to the curb. The list goes on and on.

I can't blame anyone for thinking that the heart is the most valuable player in the human body's organ inventory. After all, the heart has some well-known and established organizations acting as its publicist. Groups like the American Heart Association are always in the spotlight. Thousands of songs are written with the heart in mind. There is even a great rock band out of Seattle named Heart. To top it off, the human heart has by far the most recognizable logo on the planet: ♥ - better than Coca-Cola, McDonalds or Nike.

How can the liver compete with that?

But once the liver goes into a tailspin all hell literally breaks loose. At this point, the liver isn't the dull and boring sibling of the heart or lungs. Suddenly it's the rising star. The amount of duties that it performs is very surprising to just about everyone. Deanna and I were amazed by just how important this organ is in the body. Perhaps a major upgrade in the public relations department is needed.

In the meantime someone just has to come up with a better logo.

Chapter 12

Zachary Comes Home

For the past six weeks or so Zachary had shown enough stability to warrant discharge. But discharge for Zachary was nothing like it was for Aidan. For Aidan we simply needed a car seat and ample diapers to get us through the week. But Zachary's health needed far more hardware. He wasn't really eating much from a bottle and thus still required his food pumped into his belly. As his bowel was still in the healing mode he needed supplemental nutrients in the form of TPN and Omegaven. And since his latest surgery that separated his bowels created an ostomy he also needed a devise connected to his skin to collect the waste.

Perhaps I'm getting a little ahead of myself here. Let me back up a little and elaborate.

When Zachary underwent his latest surgical procedure the doctors had to cut away dead intestinal tissue. At this point they could have simply sewn the healthy ends of his bowel together and called it a day. However, this would eliminate the ability to physically view the condition of the bowel and thus the doctors couldn't tell if the sutured section was a healthy pink color or a less than desirable brown.

So in the meantime they allowed the top section of the intestine, or rather the part coming from the stomach to stick up through a small incision in the abdomen. This allows the docs the ability to closely monitor the condition of the bowel. As food makes its way from the belly down around the snake-like bowel to the ostomy opening it is then collected in a plastic bag attached to Zachary skin. This ostomy bag allows us to measure the amount of food and thus offers some ability to follow the efficiency of the newly tweaked bowel. It also, AND MORE IMPORTANTLY, eliminates the need for routine carpet cleaning, linen changes or overall spills of a messy nature.

After some time has passed and the doctors are comfortable with the way things are looking they reattach the two sections of intestine, suture up the abdomen and send Zachary home. This amount of time is totally arbitrary and subject to important factors like Zachary's health, his eating habits, open surgical time slots and in all probability a weekday between the hours of 7am – 3pm.

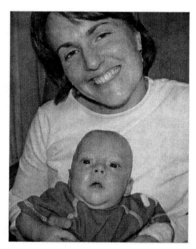

In the past Zachary would have issues like an infection or fever that made discharge impossible. But this time things started to work in his favor. Zachary's health was fine. He was tolerating minimal feeds in his belly and thus through his bowel. No fevers. No infections. Deanna and I even received training in all of his medical pumps, ostomy bags and as well as how to mix up

Zachary with Deanna

the various ingredients in his TPN & Omegaven.

On Monday February 26, 2007, after eights months of staying in the NICU, Zachary came home for the first time.

There were signs posted on our front lawn, banners across the living room picture window and balloons tethered to the mailbox. It was a great day for Zachary, for Aidan and for Deanna and myself. Let the celebration begin.

Unfortunately the celebration was short lived.

Just a few weeks later one of Zac's blood tests showed a dramatic spike in his bilirubin levels. It was high enough to suggest the beginning stages of liver failure. After much discussion and deliberation Deanna and I decided to pursue a second opinion from the folks at Johns Hopkins Medical Center also located in Baltimore. This change in venue allowed us to discuss Zachary's situation with liver and bowel specialists. They were optimistic on rehabbing his gut and had an amazing track record in doing so. The down side is that they were not a big fan of Omegaven and wanted to do away with it.

It was a tough decision but we went the Hopkins crew anyway.

Over the next several months Zachary was admitted for evaluations and over night stays. During this time we continued raising Aidan as any normal parent would. Deanna continued her part time job and took on the bulk of the household stuff while I continued to work at my full time contracting gig. With the help of aunts, uncles, grandparents and friends we found time for an occasional night out or a short kayak trip around the waters in our neighborhood.

Of course, life wasn't all fun and games. Zachary's issues took up a tremendous amount of time and since Deanna had a primo insurance plan we were allowed the use of a qualified day nurse. Keep in mind that the term "qualified" was difficult for us as parents to define. No one outside of the

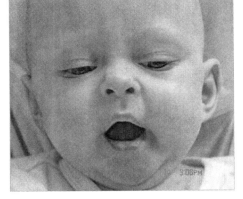

A sleepy Zachary

hospital nurses could ever measure up to our standards. But surely there could be some hint of talent in this labor pool of home nursing. Right?

The short answer is "No". The long answer is "Hell No".
Perhaps we are picky parents. Coming right out of the hospital it is
possible that we were just used to a higher standard of care. The
third option is that our instincts were right all along and that home
health care isn't what the brochures claim it to be. The correct
answer is probably a little of all three although I'm still giving more
weight to the third option.

The first home health care company was very disappointing
and was soon let go. The second company that we used had a far
superior management style but still hit-and-miss when it came to
qualified nurses. In the end we went through about twenty nurses
before we arrived at the ones we liked. Apparently finding the right
nurse it is all about volume.

Blog: Together At Last

Submitted 3/02/2007

A new page.

A new chapter.

A new beginning.

It is hard to describe what went through Deanna's and my mind as we stood in the nursery last night and finally looked upon two beautiful sleeping boys. All snuggled in their blue blankets the twins looked calm, comfortable and at ease. This would have made an excellent Norman Rockwell painting.

Of course, this didn't last too long as Aidan and Zachary are not quite on the same sleep schedule. Both boys were up for awhile during the night for no apparent reason other than to test the endurance of Mom & Dad. Hopefully we will have time to discuss the matter with the boys and make them understand how important it is to not wake up their parents. Yeah, I'm sure that this little fireside chat will set them straight. After all, we are the parents. We are the ones in charge.

Right?

We'll let everyone know how this strategy works out.

Yesterday Deanna and I absorbed a few weeks worth of medical terminology and instructions during Zachary's final day at the University of Maryland's NICU ward. Presently we are feeling a little overwhelmed by all of the information, notes and additional responsibility. Kinda like cramming for a college final exam in a course that you thought you were ready for.

Our brains are full. Give us a few days to adjust.

Brian & Deanna

Blog: Life Imitated

Submitted 3/11/2007

How I wish that life imitated our favorite tv shows. How many times did patients return to the ER under Dr. Green? How many times did Dr. House get it wrong and have to face the same sick kid? Even Dr. Quinn got it right with her antiquated and ancient medical procedures. Did any guy actually watch this show for the plot?

Every sick patient got better! Every sick patient went home for good...never to return again! We liked these writers. They gave us a sense of calm and upbeatness. Unfortunately Zachary's script was written by different people.

Zac's weekly blood test showed some disturbing readings associated with his liver. How disturbing? Well, they were scary enough for us to face more hospital time with little hesitation. After eight months of prior hospital residency at UMMS one can probably get a feeling just how much we really wanted to avoid this situation.

Okay, so here is the current situation: Zachary is now at Johns Hopkins Medical Center (Baltimore, MD) in the pediatric ward. He was admitted last Friday after a lengthy consult with one of their most experienced doctors. Deanna and I were convinced that our home health approach wasn't doing him any favors and that admitting him was the best thing for him.

The doctors...specialists in this area of trouble boast quite abit of experience. They have been incredibly helpful in explaining the situation from their perspective and what their game plan is in getting Zachary back to better health. From what I can tell it seems like a good game plan. Of course, the pre-game show is not always the same as the post-game show.

Realistically the medical folks have to take a few days to become familiar with Zac's medical history and this alone is no easy task. The paper supply alone probably *took out half of the trees in Washington State. Personally I would have waited for the movie.*

Still, the folks in white lab coats exude confidence and have a pretty impressive track record in this sort of thing. In the meantime Deanna and myself will alternate night duties so our son will not have to go without Mommy or Daddy. It may be inconvenient for us but imagine how he feels. More alarms. More buzzers. More needles.

Yuck!

Brian & Deanna

Blog: Yellow Hospital Gowns

Submitted 4/06/2007

Not too long ago when Zachary was in the NICU we would make the daily trip to the hospital. We endured the arduous task of finding a parking space in the nearby parking garage, walking past the US Smoking Team tryouts in the heavily posted "No Smoking Zone", waiting for the extremely slow elevators to take us up to the 6th floor and finally wearing those incredibly ugly banana colored gowns just to have the joy and pleasure of holding our son.

One does a lot for a smile and eye contact with your child.

Now that Zachary is home one would think that the hard part is behind us. WRONG! We no longer have the luxury of heading to our home at the end of the evening and leaving the monitoring of medicines and feed to the wonderful NICU nurses. (If there is one thing that we can never overemphasis is the depth of talent in these nurses.)

Now it is us who have to monitor his food intake, waste output, temperature readings, program pumps, change IV tubes, check for dehydration, check for rehydration, analyze diaper usage, empty ostomy bags, stock supplies and finally manage the barrage of home health nurses that come into your home to care for our son.

Finding the right home health care nurse is like searching for the Holy Grail. It is elusive, requires hard work and downright difficult to do without some trial and error. Take for instance our saga.

We started off with a company that camed highly recommended. In hindsight, we should have skipped over this recommendation. This company sent out a handful of nurses to care for Zachary - only one really was of any quality. The others required our constant attention as we never fully let our guard down. This is provided, of course, that they even showed up for their shift. Ah, don't get me started!

This company was fired the other day.

We are now with company #2. So far there is a 1000% increase in professionalism and the nurses ask lots of questions and seem far more prepared. They even showed up on time! As parents, our guard is still up and perhaps this will recede soon...maybe. We are kinda winging it at the moment.

So the bottom line is that the grass isn't always greener outside of the NICU but then again, we don't have to wear ugly banana colored hospital gowns either.

Brian & Deanna

Chapter 13

Getting On With Our Lives

A s we approached the twin's first birthday on July 2, 2007 Deanna and I had a few opportunities to sit back and reflect on our lives since Zachary was discharged from UMMS back on February 26th. There were many emotional ups and downs as well as optimistic highs and...shall I say optimistic not so highs. During this time period we had to admit Zachary in and out of Johns Hopkins so many times that I ended up losing count. But through this whole process, no matter how dark and dreary it appeared we never lost our motivation of having our family together under one roof.

We were committed (or arguably should have been committed) to get Zachary home no matter what. We would never look back a decade from now and wonder if we could have tried harder. Planning for the future could wait for now. It was more important to live in the present. Throughout it all I would say that we were keeping our sanity in check, sort of. Who knew that this was the easy part?

The twins' first birthday party was a raging success. The sky was sunny and the weather was beautiful. It was a full house inside and out. A huge variety of food was available on a large table all contained in stainless steel tubs separated by colorful balloons. One of Zachary's NICU nurse's husband had a side business setting up inflatable bouncy castle thing-a-ma-jigs. It was the sort of attraction that all the kids (and many adults) had to enter and romp around for a while. During the party, Aidan was the center of attention but it was Zachary who was the star attraction. So many friends, family and neighbors showed up to celebrate this amazing year.

A few days later on July 5th Zachary was once again admitted into Johns Hopkins for his highly anticipated reanastomosis (huge fancy word for the bowel reconnection) operation. Unlike the other emergency surgeries in the past, this procedure was planned and important to note, planned AFTER the birthday party. No way was another operation interfering with Aidan & Zachary's one-year birthday party.

The reconnection of the bowel was necessary for Zachary's recovery. At this point it all becomes a game of Dominoes. A connected bowel means that there is more length of tissue to absorb his digested food. The extra-absorbed food means more vital nutrients in the body and thus less dependence on TPN & Omegaven. This lessened dependence will eventually equate to a stronger liver and finally, a stronger liver allows for a healthier Zachary.

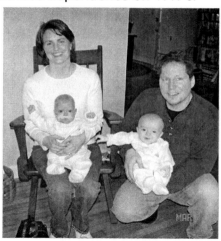

The operation went very well and after three weeks of recovery time Zachary was home once again resuming a life outside of the hospital.

Of course we knew beforehand that if the bowel didn't end up absorbing the nutrients as hoped then Zachary would continue to be

First family photo at home.

dependent on TPN & Omegaven. Although we had high hopes for success, the medical prognosis prepared us ahead of time for a different possibility.

For the next few weeks we continued with our daily routines. We fed Zachary, walked around the neighborhood with the twins and for all practical purposes continued our lives with optimism and high hopes. But after a few weeks the doctors told us that in spite of the reanastomosis his blood tests continued to show disappointing results. In all likelihood his liver may continue to trend downward.

They suggested that we get a consultation with a leading liver / bowel transplant specialist before things got worse. The question was which specialist? There are a handful of these qualified centers throughout the country ranging from locations like Miami, Omaha, Los Angeles, Georgetown (DC) and Pittsburgh. Ultimately we decided that the center in Pittsburgh, PA was the most experienced and had the longest and most successful track record. It was considered by many to be one of the best in the country, if not the world. It wasn't the closest location from our house but at a five-hour drive north it was manageable.

We had set up the initial meeting a few weeks out with the team at Children's Hospital of Pittsburgh. Deanna had gathered all of Zachary's pertinent medical information in an overflowing binder and was ready to discuss his health and possible transplant with the doctors. We were soon to be in a whole new realm of medical science. Not to worry though as we had a few weeks to study the new terms.

Life had other plans for us.

A week later Zachary took a turn for the worse.

On Sunday we noticed the Zac was sleeping more. Perhaps he was catching up on some sleep, perhaps he was going through a healing phase, perhaps this, perhaps that. We came to the conclusion that someone with a MD after their name needed to look at him.

The next day we decided to take Zachary up to the Pediatric Emergency Room at Johns Hopkins. On route he still looked sleepy and lethargic which was all very concerning. When my nudges and light slaps on his face produced no effects I asked Deanna to speed up, run a few lights and get there faster. After the doctors did their analysis he was promptly admitted to the ICU.

The lab results were numerous ranging from high ammonia levels (204), high bilirubin (29), low platelet count (10), etc... Basically he was in shock and experiencing liver failure. Not quite the news a parent wants to hear. We were told that if we had not brought him up at this time then the outcome...(dramatic pause by the doctor)...would have been very bad. I think we understood what wasn't said.

Several days went by and things just didn't get better. He was too fragile to fly to Pittsburgh for a transplant and even if he was, there was no guarantee that organs would be available. It was up to the doctors at Johns Hopkins to buy his body more time. It was a lot to ask but ask we did. For the next few days Zachary barely held his own. We watched in amazement how such a little guy could take on so much and fight for his very survival. His blood pressure was weak, his kidneys were slowing down and his body had absorbed so much fluid that he soon resembled the Michelin man. And if this wasn't enough there were now signs of an infection. Things just didn't look good.

For the next several days we watched some ups and some downs - always hovering around the same level of instability. However, ten days later things changed. Zachary continued to show some improvement in several areas like blood pressure, heart rate as well as breathing conditions. So many other areas were monitored that frankly, no one without an advanced degree in medicine could possibly remember it all.

But the big question I asked was simple: Was Zachary able to be transported to Pittsburgh? The answer was a resounding "Maybe". The Hopkins docs were waiting for some improvements in his health to make his flight easier as well as to give him a better standing as a transplant candidate. Some of these improvements that they spoke of were not exactly what I expected. You see, your standing on the transplant list is like trying to get into Harvard – you need a good score. But the mathematics to this calculation include some sort of an X factor understood only by medical trained personnel.

Here is how this works. The sicker Zachary was means that he is more likely to get placed at the top of the list, hence he may get organs sooner. On the other side of the coin, the healthier Zachary was means that he would be placed a little farther down the list and thus may have to wait for organs. So the docs want to get him healthy...but not to healthy. Understand?

If this concept wasn't enough to grasp, we heard that no matter what the outcome was we couldn't fly Zachary to Pittsburgh anyway. The reason was simply because Children's had no room available. All of their PICU (Pediatric Intensive Care Unit) beds were full and there were actually potential patients on some sort of PICU stand-by list. Kinda brings back memories on how Deanna and myself could not find a hospital to take the twins at delivery. So in the meantime Deanna and I juggled Zac's needs with Aidan's needs – our needs of course were put on hold. There was a lot going on and unfortunately this was only the beginning.

Blog: Debating Skills

Submitted 5/05/2007

At the last posting we were in the mindset that Zachary's reconnection of the ostomies was gonna happen in the near future.

We were eager. We were confident. We were wrong.

After some recent conversations with the Hopkins team we felt that we made the case for Zac's reconnection. We threw in terms like "quality of life" and "physical development". Mighty powerful arguments we thought. We basked in our debating skills.

With this perfectly maneuvered verbal power play, the GI doctor hopped on board with this process and referred us to make an appointment with the surgeon. Yippee! The surgeon discussed the matter with us and he too was on board with the surgery. Yippee again! Now here is where I get lost in the medical rationale.

Apparently after the surgeon started sharpening up his Ginsu operating knives, Zac had his weekly blood test which showed a dramatic improvement in his liver condition from the previous week. Let me reiterate: Dramatic Improvement. At this point, the GI doctor reintervened and wanted to postpone the surgery in hope that continued liver improvement would happen. Continued improvement meant limiting the risk of liver complications during the surgery.

So if I understand this correctly: the surgery was okay when his liver was in decent shape. But when the liver got better the surgery became riskier. And to reduce risk, we have to wait until the liver becomes healthier.

????????

This is why I was a business major. The new game plan is now to wait about another three weeks to reevaluate. Arrrrgh!

Please stay tuned for more updates on "The Life and Times of Zachary's Liver Related Blood Readings".

Followed by "The Stress Levels of the Johnson Household" playing at a theater near you.

Brian & Deanna

Blog: A Few More Bottles

Submitted 07/05/2007

"Lower Stress Levels" for $1000 please.
No more intestines sticking out of the stomach.
No more ostomy bags.
No more tubes sticking out through a nose.
What is a "Successful Reanastomosis Operation" Alex.

Yes, it is true! The operation - Zac's sixth overall since birth, was successful. Let the Happy Hour begin! Let's all belly up to the bar and toast for the little guy.

It all began this morning as Deanna, Zachary, and I drove the 30 minute commute to Johns Hopkins for his surgical prep. After some blood draws and some Q&A from the surgical staff he was wheeled away by doctors in blue scrubs. Nothing to do now but wait.

They tell you to relax in the waiting room and one does everything but that. Somewhere during this exercise in futility we decided to have a one star luncheon at the cafeteria. Eh, one star might be pushing it.

Anyway, after three hours the lead surgeon found us flipping through some old magazines and after finding some quiet space in a noisy hallway, gave us the optimal news.

Now we can spend somewhat of a relaxing night with Deanna's folks, Aidan and a few more bottles of unopened wine.

Now where is that corkscrew?

Brian & Deanna

Blog: *Waiting for a Bed*

Submitted 08/21/2007

As of Tuesday Zachary was holding his own in the Pediatric ICU. His blood pressure, breathing rate and heart rate isn't stellar material but within acceptable levels. His liver is pretty much on the final turn and the intestines are not really helping matters much. There are hints of an infection (i.e. elevated white blood count) yet no blood cultures are showing positive signs. Odd huh.

When the docs feel that he is stable enough for the air ride he will be flown to Pittsburgh where he will await a liver/bowel transplant. This may take awhile (hurry up and wait) but we feel that it is important to get him up there ASAP anyway. So we are trying to get Zachary transported to Children's Hospital of Pittsburgh when a bed becomes available.

Yep, can you believe this? In spite of everything Zac has gone through we are now in a position of waiting for a bed to become available. One can't make this kinda stuff up.

So the bottom line is that we called the PICU nurse 10 minutes ago for an update. Now we are going to bed. I suspect we will call at 3am for another update and will do so again at 6:30. It is tough to sleep at night with this looming over our heads.

Of course, think of how Zachary feels. Suddenly my sleep schedule really doesn't matter that much.

Brian & Deanna

Blog: Bag of Bananas

Submitted 08/28/2007

Zachary continues to show stability in his current situation. Because he ballooned up so much in the past week, the staff is constantly monitoring his net fluid intake, potassium and ammonia levels, breathing conditions and so many other areas that frankly, no non-medical human could possibly remember it all.

As parents, Deanna and I sit by Zac's bed to comfort, to stare and to hope. We wonder just how many times an infant can rebound from such evasive procedures. You gotta admit that the human body is truly an amazing organism.

For instance, I'm told that his body regulates potassium levels. Really? I had no idea that what I ate had potassium. How many times does someone feel low potassium levels and runs out to the late night banana bar at Denny's to stock up on this nutrient? When I was told of his ammonia level all I could think of was that blue colored stuff in Windex.

Even through the intense learning curve that I have experienced in this past 14 months I have come to the conclusion that I will never fully understand the intricacies of the human body. My medical knowledge is contained to areas such as aspirin, chapstick and band-aids. At 43 I'm pretty sure that medical school isn't in the cards so in the meantime I will grab a doctor and ask my questions.

So for now we wait for the swelling to go down, the ammonia levels to return to normal and the potassium percentage to reduce. Perhaps I'll buy a bag of bananas just in case!

Brian & Deanna

Chapter 14

The Flight to Pittsburgh

From the outside looking in our lives were full of uncertainty and stress. After all, we had a young son laying in a pediatric ICU whose life was hanging by a thread. By all accounts, Deanna and I should be chain smoking and doing shots of hard liquor along with daily therapy sessions with the local psychologist. But somehow we developed a routine that allowed for work, hospital visits, grocery shopping, doggy walks as well as raising Aidan.

This routine was about to change.

On September 1, 2007 I had just arrived back at the house following a three-hour visit at the Hopkins ICU. As I was shutting the screen door I heard the phone ring. It was the Hopkins ICU doctors stating that a bed had become

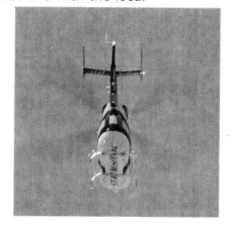

Life Flight to Children's

available at the Children's PICU in Pittsburgh. "Great news" I replied. "We'll be up in the morning to see him off." "If you want the bed space we need to leave now" was her response. "You mean now...as in tonight?" "Now...as in the helicopter pilot is waiting on the launch pad" she added.

At 7pm Zachary left Johns Hopkins Medical Center helipad on a non-stop flight for Pittsburgh.

At that point it was a matter of logistics for there were a lot of decisions and preparations to do before leaving the next morning.

In the meantime we would coordinate baby-sitting services with Deanna's parents – not sure how long. Our pets would have to be cared for by someone – not sure who. We needed to pack – not sure how much. After all, who knows how long we will be out of town. It could be a few days. It could be a few weeks. Pittsburgh is kinda close to our house in Severna Park but not THAT close. I wish I could say that we could rely on some sort of prior similar experience to draw upon. Alas, this was not the case. We were in the "fly by the seat of your pants" mode.

Full steam ahead.

The next day we left early. With a full tank of gas, toll quarters and a map we were ready for the five hour drive to Pittsburgh. We discussed Zachary's health. We discussed where we would live. We discussed how Aidan and our trusted hound Bailey would stay with Deanna's parents in nearby Cleveland during this process. It didn't take long – a few hours at best that we realized that we were done planning. It was time to veg out and turn on the radio. There would be plenty of time to talk about our lives and how it revolved around Zachary. If only we knew just how much of an understatement that actually was.

Chapter 15

Welcome to Children's Hospital of Pittsburgh

I lived in Cleveland for about seven years in the 90's and Deanna grew up in nearby Chardon located just a half hour east. Living on the North Coast we learned to appreciate the diversity of the city, we learned to tolerate the bitter winters and above all else, we learned to dislike Pittsburgh. It's a football aspect. You know, the Browns vs. the Steelers - the whole rust belt rivalry thing. Thankfully the Keystone border patrol didn't take that into consideration when we crossed the state line into Pennsylvania.

We arrived at Children's Hospital at around 2 pm that day. Between the use of a map, the various Pittsburgh road signs and Map Quest we were able to successfully navigate right up and into the wrong parking garage. In spite of the early blunder we were

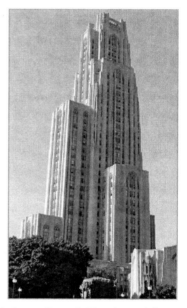

University of Pittsburgh's Cathedral of Learning

able to find the hospital, the PICU and of course Zachary who was resting comfortably in Bed 15. Even though he was in a new location, he was just like when we left him at Hopkins - laying peacefully and fully sedated with a ventilator tube in his mouth. It all seemed so surreal, like we were in the audience watching a movie. But reality is not always a pleasant thing as we were reminded by the ever present blinking and buzzing monitors. How long would this movie last?

It wasn't long before the PICU doctors met with us to begin discussing Zachary's condition. I suspect that this first meeting was more for our benefit as the Hopkins' crew did a thorough job of relaying Zachary's condition. The Children's PICU attending doctor asked us several questions and then outlined her assessment of the situation. There wasn't a lot of new information for us to absorb. Most of which we knew from the past 12 months of hospital visits. But we were here for different reasons. Zachary needed new organs. That we knew. When this would happen was still anyone's guess.

In the meantime we had coordinated the handoff of Aidan (along with our dog Bailey) to Deanna's folks. They would be in charge of spoiling their grandson (and grand dog) for a week or two until Mom and Dad became acclimated to their new surroundings. For now we would focus on Zachary and arrange for some overnight accommodations throughout this ordeal.

Most hospitals have a social worker whose job, among many others, is to help parents like us find somewhere to sleep. The options range from expensive to cheap. We opted for the cheap. After a few nights of sleeping at a friend's spare bedroom we arranged for a longer stay at the Ronald McDonald House located in the nearby Shadyside district. We had a small room in a beautiful Victorian home complete with a shared kitchen, Internet service and a wonderful staff who made our stay as pleasant as possible. Located just a few miles from the hospital, we could zip in at any time of the day or night to check in on our son.

By this time Aidan had returned to our fold. Throughout the next few weeks and months the three us became more familiar with Pittsburgh and all that it had to offer. I gotta admit that all of the Cleveland propaganda was entirely wrong. Pittsburgh is an amazing city with lots to see and do as well as sporting a distinct family friendly flair. There are lots of parks and playgrounds in and near the Shadyside district. A short walk from the hospital is a very impressive Museum of Natural History, the Phipps Botanical Garden as well as several libraries that cater to both adults and children. If you take Zachary's issues out of the equation, we would actually be enjoying our visit to Pittsburgh.

Within a week of our arrival in Pittsburgh we had seen some small improvements in Zachary health. His water weight had shown some reduction, his dependence on blood pressure medications had lessened and many of his electrolytes started to stabilize. But sometimes, no matter how hard Zachary's body tries to get better there were always obstacles. Of course this is a lesson that we learned early and was reminded often. Because of these obstacles we would be introduced to a plethora of machines intended to either mimic or compliment the human body.

There were ventilators and oscillators that helped Zachary to breathe. There were dialysis pumps that cycled and filtered his blood. There were tanks filled with oxygen and helium intended to balance chemicals in his lungs. There was a space heater of sorts that blew warm air into a plastic blanket just to keep Zachary's temperature at a normal level. And when Zachary's temperature was too high, the use of a simple fan was turned on.

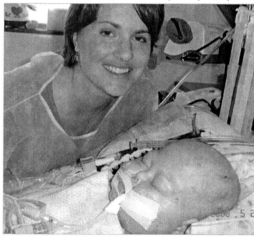

Deanna with Zachary (post transplant)

Sometimes the amount of machines crowded out any free space near Zachary's crib and thus moved our chairs out to an uncomfortable distance from our son. Sometimes it was a tight squeeze just to stand at arm's length of Zachary. Who knew that there were so many apparatuses in connection with the PICU? I often wondered just how large the room was that housed all of this equipment. From the likes of how many machines Zachary needed, it most have been a large room.

For the first three months of Zachary's stay he lay on his back. Fully sedated and immobilized was our son. It was not an easy thing for a parent to view day in and day out. You want to see progress. You desire something, anything really to show that your child is getting better. What we had to accept was that progress is not always measurable by monitors and rulers. In fact, Zachary needed a hefty amount of drugs just to keep him stable and that in itself was something to be thankful for. We realized soon enough that we needed to change our definition of progress and change it daily.

But try as we could, we could never define progress – at least not on a daily basis. Yes, we knew that the big picture involved a transplant and eventual discharge from the hospital. But in the interim our way of thinking was much different. At times, many times actually, there were improvements in Zachary's health. It is only natural for us to get excited but experience taught us that we had to temper our emotions. After all, there were so many times that Deanna and I have seen the sudden downfall of Zachary's improvements. It seems to be the law of averages that our son has adhered to throughout his short life. Even though we should keep up some type of emotional guard, we usually faltered and fell asleep that night hoping for the best – or rather more than the best. After all, he is our son. This is what parents do.

Throughout Zachary's time in the PICU he was constantly barraged by infections. This is considered a swear word of sorts in this setting – one that you NEVER want connected with a patient. Certainly not with a patient hanging onto life and especially not with a patient who is on the transplant list. When a transplant candidate gets an infection they are pretty much taken off of the transplant list. This window of opportunity for available organs is short enough – you don't want to reduce it any more with infections. But the sad truth is that sick kids in the hospital tend to get infections more frequently for the simple fact that they are in the hospital. There is no better place to catch a virus.

Everyday, it seemed, we were thrown yet another curve. Whether it was an infection, electrolyte imbalance or low blood pressure something was always awry. No matter what time of day it seemed that we were always on the tips of our toes. But the curves, as it turned out, were not limited to Zachary alone.

Sometime around the month of January 2008, Deanna informed me that lately she just wasn't feeling right. She stated that she was more tired than usual and added that in addition; she was a month late with her menstrual cycle. "Perhaps I'm pregnant", she mumbled jokingly.

Now I consider myself an average Joe of sorts. I can operate a circular saw in a somewhat confident fashion. I can chalk a cue stick like the next guy and when pressed I can whip up an impressive pan of scrabbled eggs. Throughout my life I feel that I can, if needed, take control of a situation with an aura of leadership. So when my wife hinted at the possibility of another baby in the pipeline I quickly jumped into presidential mode.

I reminded her that the twins were the result of many years of natural attempts followed by daily injections of hormone drugs followed by an expensive route of Petri dish speed dating. The result was that we spent over $12K on obtaining two children. "Rest assured" I said, "There is absolutely no way that you are pregnant." A few days later the blood test came back.

It turns out that I was wrong.

Apparently, it took 17 months of daily hospital visits as well as large amounts of added stress to start the pregnancy train rolling in full motion. Looking back, we didn't have to go through all of the drugs and financial expenses after all. The more I thought of it, the more I wanted our money back.

The fact that another child would soon be upon us was a nice distraction but a temporary one at that. We still had to deal with the important aspect of a son in the hospital. So whatever the health of Zachary we continued with our routines. Part of the day Deanna was at his crib and the other part of the day I was. Throughout this time period Aidan continued to grow up, crawl, walk and play with toys. We had our three meals a day and followed Zachary's progress like full time medical students.

But try as we might, it was not easy to rise above the stress of the situation. The daytime hours, it seems, were a little easier on our nerves. At that time of the day one of us could sit by Zachary's crib and often discuss his cares with the doctors. Even if we did nothing it still provided us with the sense that our presence helped and in some way nudged Zachary along for another day.

However, when the night shift came around our plan hit a compromise. We felt that we needed to hang out with Aidan at our apartment and continue some semblance of family life. It also meant much needed sleep for Deanna and myself. This of course ultimately translated into more time away from Zachary.

It seemed to be an unfair compromise but it was the best plan on the books. Even though we were away from Zachary our minds were always on him.

Would our son make it through the night and see the next morning? Would the phone ring in the middle of the night with bad news? We tried not to think such thoughts but optimism carries only so much weight. At times your duties as a worrying parent take center stage. This proved to be a constant battle of emotions that was at times very draining on mind, body and soul.

This was how we lived our lives during this first seven months of Zachary's stay at Children's.

Blog: Mass Transit

Submitted 09/06/2007

Zachary's condition seems to be trending in a positive direction. Albeit a slow trend, it is positive nevertheless.

So many of his labs results continue the yo-yo methodology (a medical term). For instance, one day his potassium level is up and the next it is down. The same goes for magnesium, calcium, ammonia, platelets, hemoglobin levels, etc... After I get a look at the morning blood results I realize that I have no idea what any of this means.

Still, I rub my chin like I have a firm grasp on the situation and say things like "hmm" or "interesting". I got this idea from watching the doctors on General Hospital.

Currently Deanna and I have obtained short-term housing at the Ronald McDonald house in the Shadyside area of Pittsburgh. It is a beautiful and very large Victorian house with lots of bedrooms (we are in #34), three kitchens, and laundry facilities...basically alot like our house in Severna Park, MD (yes, that would be sarcasm).

This residence is right next to the main bus line that stops next to Children's Hospital. Taking the bus seemed like a no brainer - fast and efficient. Mass transit at its best. Of course, this idea also resonates with about 2000 other University of Pittsburgh students.

So here we were yesterday - just Deanna, myself and 400 of our closest new friends all crammed together so close I could hear their eyes blink. What does one say to another when my elbow repeatedly jams into their ribs or when I stepped on someone's feet and couldn't move away due to the sardine factor? What is the proper etiquette here?

Today we drove!

Brian & Deanna

Blog: *Mannerisms*

Submitted 09/09/2007

It is no secret that Zachary is at Children's Hospital for a liver / small bowel transplant. However, upon his arrival he had slid backwards a tad and was deemed too sick to list for transplant.

Too Sick?

Wasn't this the very reason for the trip to PA? Well, after the docs explained that they needed an infection free Zachary with stable blood pressure it all made sense. So finally, after nine days of PICU care, our little lad is starting to fit the desired mold. His blood pressure is looking better, his water weight is being shed and he is getting some stability in his essential electrolytes. These Pittsburgh doctors are pretty smart! Not only are they getting Zachary stable but they have to convey this information to the parents.

It's odd how many of these doctors use the same mannerisms when giving a medical prognosis to parents. It seems to be the same methodology across many of the institutions that we have associated. Perhaps Medical Communication 101?

For instance:
Action: Doctor enters room.

Mannerism: Doctor usually carries clipboard or other medical chart.
Reason: This gives some authority to their presence.
Statement: "Mr. & Mrs. Johnson, I have the results of Zachary's lab test".

Mannerism: Doctor folds arms in a slow fashion and begins a gentle yet standing rocking motion.
Reason: Two theories really:

1) The rocking motion stimulates blood flow which allows clearer thought patterns and increased communication skills.
2) Doctor is breaking in some new shoes.

Mannerism: *Doctor glances up at light fixture, breathes deep and exhales while gently unfolding arms. Clip board is usually held with right hand at hip position.*
Reason: *This is the most non threatening position for mammals (watch Animal Planet for further documentation). It allows the doctor to present good or bad news to the now sweat drenched parents.*

Mannerism: *Doctor reads off some lab results and looks at resident or intern as if to validate his/her conclusion. Intern searches frantically through notes for some clue of doctor's intention. Of course, only the doctor knows that it takes years of experience to perfect this body language. Doctor then turns to parents for direct eye contact thus letting intern off the hook. A slight tap of the left foot further enhances authority.*
Reason: *Doctor is setting the stage for direct verbal communication.*

Mannerism: *Doctor places clipboard down on bedside and places pen in lab coat pocket (clicking of pen is optional).*
Reason: *Doctor is getting ready to present medical situation and game plan for solution. This series of carefully crafted gestures help to hypnotize parents into listening with 100% concentration. Without this ceremonious assortment of movements, many parents would be distracted by the many alarms and noises often associated with hospital rooms.*

So there you have it! I have cracked to doctor - patient/parent code! Feel free to use this knowledge with all further doctor visits, parent-teacher conferences and when arguing with police over speeding tickets.

Brian & Deanna

Blog: Confuse the Doctors

Submitted 09/13/2007

There are two confusing aspects of Zachary's stay here at Children's. One is his ability to confuse the doctors and the other is the ability of the doctors to confuse me.

Take for instance the latest 24 hours:

Doctors: Zachary has lost over a liter of fluids over the past day.

Brian: Wow! That is good news.

Doctors: No, not really. We don't want him to lose too much weight this quickly or as you can see, his blood pressure has dropped a little too much. Zachary is a challenging case so we will cut his diuretic somewhat and put him on a small amount of dopamine to counter this effect.

Brian: Yes, I understand that. The dopamine will constrict the blood vessels and thus raise his blood pressure. So increasing this drug will in the future will solve this dilemma. So this is a step in the right direction.?

Doctors: No, not really. Relying on this drug is a band aid approach. We really need Zachary to do this on his own. However, we are having trouble figuring him out. If the blood pressure increases too much we may opt to lower the steroids that he is currently on.

Brian: Oh, I see now. So the bottom line is to adjust the steroids, which will affect the vessels, blood flow and overall health of my son. So when the blood pressure is low, then raising the steroids is a good thing.

Doctors: No, that is a bad thing. Steroids really are a last resort approach. Instead we may decide to increase the albumin level for Zachary. This will help draw fluid from his tissues into the blood stream. Hopefully this will help in the long-term approach.

Brian: Ah, how silly of me to think otherwise. So giving Zachary albumin is the approach. So in the future you can just give him this blood product and everything will fall in line. Finally, a good thing.

Doctors: No, albumin is synthesized by the liver. This is why he needs a transplant.

 Basically I decided to shut up and direct all questions to Deanna.
 If you have questions about Zac's condition, don't ask me...ask Deanna.

Brian

Blog: Behavior Psychiatrist

Submitted 09/16/2007

 Zachary's condition has mystified many a medical personnel ranging from surgical doctors at the University of Maryland Medical Center, the GI doctors at Johns Hopkins and finally the ICU doctors at Children's. Yes, everyone agreed that the liver was failing and everyone is on board with the bowel not absorbing nutrients. But there was and still is something else going on that causes Zac to drop his blood pressure or have issues with his breathing or any of a dozen so or more problems.

Keep in mind that Pittsburgh has had over 1200 liver & small bowel transplants. The ICU doc told us that Zac was probably in his top 5 of all the problem kiddie patients. Not exactly a positive statistic that I want embroidered on his afghan baby blanket. Still, we are here for a transplant and we have to jump through a number of hoops in this program.

Take for instance our required meeting with the Behavior Psychiatrist this past week. Apparently the medical staff feels the need to screen the parents to insure that they are up for the long and arduous task of parenting a transplantee. In fact, they require this hour long meeting so the shrink can size up mom and dad and provide some sort of feedback to the transplant committee.

We met with this fella and was asked several questions. Make sure you slow down the speed of the questions to get the full effect like:

1. "How...do you feel...about Zachary's...condition?"
2. "How...are you...handling the...stress?"
3. "How do you...get by each day...with bad...news?"

Really, I'm not making any of this up!

Yeah, we answered the questions in a professional way but the real answers involved something along the lines of banging your head, early happy hour and extreme sarcasm on a Carepage web site. Either way, this required meeting amounted to a huge waste of time and further confirmed the probability that Deanna and I will soon be admitted to a mental institution for full evaluation.

Still, was this formal evaluation feedback in some sort of written form or something more basic like the following:

Zachary Johnson's Parents (check one)
____ *Sane*
____ *Insane*

I'll keep everyone posted on our mental score when they arrive.

Brian & Deanna

Blog: City Slickers
Submitted 9/21/2007

Anyone remember the 1991 movie City Slickers? There is a scene where the three main characters are herding cows over a vast prairie. The main character, Billy Crystal is attempting to explain to his buddy how to program a vcr. After several attempts of explaining this process over several hours his friend could never grasp the concept.

This is how I felt when the nurse tried to explain the CVVH machine to me. She talked about fluids going in and how they were extracted. She talked about net differences and how Zac's urine figures were calculated in the equation. She mentioned non-calculated figures and how this somehow factored into it all.

Positives & Negatives.
Intakes & Outtakes.
Pluses and Minuses.
Blah blah blah.

I asked several questions - many twice. And in the end I felt like the cowboy on the prairie...I just didn't get it. Zachary got it. The Amish kid two beds down got it. Some of the homeless guys near the hospital may have gotten wind of it. But not me.

But hey, as long as the nurses understand it! That's the important thing.

Brian & Deanna

Blog: Asking Questions

Submitted 09/23/2007

When we first arrived at Children's we were ushered into the Pediatric ICU and shown where Zachary would be spending some time at Bed 15. We met his night nurse and was given a pretty good overall explanation of his situation and what to expect within the next 24 hours. At this time we heard what would be a very familiar statement uttered by all people connected with Zac's care:

"Don't hesitate to ask any questions."

In the past three weeks or so Zac has seen a few dozen or so nurses, a handful of attending doctors, 6 fellows, scores of residents and I lots and lots of respiratory therapists. So in the past month we have had a large spectrum of medical personal to pose questions, obtain clarification and further explain some of the intricacies of Zac's medical conditions. Compliment this with a wide assortment of "what if" scenarios and other questions that started with "if you had to guess...".

No one says anything about asking questions anymore!

My thought is that word has spread among the medical staff to stay the hell away from Bed #15. But Zachary's corner area is like a black hole - it draws them in for the inevitable question. Hey, can I help it if I want further clarification on how may red blood cells are created by Zachary in both a sick and healthy state? Or when exactly did syringes change from glass to plastic? Why is it that only the doctors wear the white lab coats?

Yes, the questions are many and the answers are amazingly articulated. Strangely enough, many of these questions actually have something to do with Zachary. And hey, it's not our fault that we ask so many questions. If the ICU concierge had put us in a location that had a tv then we would be too distracted watching reruns of MacGyver.

Instead, we ask questions.

Brian & Deanna

Blog: *An International Team*

Submitted 09/26/2007

During our three week visit at Children's, we have been besieged by doctors for the transplant team. So far, there have been eight or so that I can remember.

The main doctor is sorta like a soap opera doctor. He is experienced, gray haired and has a presence that emulates confidence. I would say that if a movie was made about him then I would pick Charleston Heston to be his actor. Yes, the man who played Moses and wrested with the apes would be a great pick.

The second doctor has similar features in that he has some graying around the temples, uses big medical terms and tends to stop his sentence structure as if searching for the best possible combination of words for the most accurate portrayal of his thoughts. Probably a Harvard grad! I would pick Alan Alda for his actor. How can a man with a cool nickname who saved hundreds of lives during the Korean War be a bad pick?

The third doctor spoke with a distinct Australian accent. I fully expected him to invite me out to the local reptile farm to weigh and tag the lizards. For his actor would be no other than Crocodile Dundee). Eh mate?

Ah, an international team! Now what could be better than that? A group of doctors combining knowledge of medicine based on years of experience from around the globe.

This is where the comparison felt kinda short.

The next doctor that I met was an anesthesiologist. He was young...very young. I mean, it's not like I expect every doctor involved in Zachary's care to have voted in the 1972 election but can we at least stay away from doctors who are actively using Clearasil? I want a doctor who looks more like Ward than the Beaver.

I'll admit that I am not being totally fair here but as a parent we have an obligation if not a right to err slightly on the side of emotion. It was in the Bill or Rights...somewhere towards the back!

Either way you look at it, younger or older, the Children's transplant team will be excellent. We'll let you know when "Zachary Johnson, The Movie" premieres to a theater near you.

Brian & Deanna

Blog: Steeler Sunday

Submitted 09/27/2007

Upon entering the PICU the other day we walked to Zachary's crib like we do every other time. We make a straight bee line and sorta not look at any of the other patients. Whether they be left or right, port or starboard, proper etiquette, it seems, is to concentrate on your child and not on anyone else's. Well, being an open floor plan at Children's it is a tad difficult to follow this rule but one has to admit that life in general kinda grooms you for this.

Take for instance when you enter an auto dealership at lunch time. There are approximately three hundred people on the sale force tripping over themselves trying to sell you a car. The rule of thumb is simple: Look straight ahead and no matter what: DON'T MAKE EYE CONTACT!

The same rules apply when a guy spots an ex-girlfriend at a restaurant with his wife at his side. Arguably there is usually a wrong way and a right way to handle this but in all reality the best approach is simple: Stare at your feet at all times and no matter what: DON'T MAKE EYE CONTACT!

So it wasn't so hard to keep with the PICU rules when visiting Zachary. But after a few weeks of bee line mentality I noticed my eyes may have wandered outside of the approved zone. It occurred to me one Sunday that I had some company in this laxed attitude. Of course, it wasn't that the other parents didn't care about their little girl Sally as much as they found the Steelers game on their crib side tv a tad more interesting.

Have I ever mentioned that Zac has no tv at his crib?

I then noticed that there were several doctors and other medical types hanging out in the PICU doing what appeared to be...well, absolutely nothing. They too were fixated on the tv surrounding everyone's crib (well, not Zachary's of course) and from time to time, usually during commercials, would make some sort of notation on the patient's form.

I learned later that the PICU was the only place at Children's Hospital that had televisons. Not sure if this was good thing but you gotta admit that if anything had happened to Zachary then there were plenty of medical brains standing around to help.

Well, as long as it was halftime.

Brian & Deanna

Blog: Second Hand Smoke

Submitted 09/29/2007

Ask anyone and they will tell you that hospitals are not an enjoyable place to visit. Designers have tried to compensate by adopting the shopping center approach with features like a water fountain, Starbucks and a cookie kiosk. Eh, it's a start.

Not to long ago there used to be dozens of smokers standing outside of the hospital entrance at Children's getting their nicotine fix. This provided a negative impression to the visitor and a solution was needed. To solve this problem about twenty "No Smoking" signs were posted from the entrance to the street.

Of course this worked about as well as Oktoberfest in Chinatown. Upon entering from the street most every visitor will get their Surgeon General's recommended amount of second hand smoke. According to our high school algebra calculations, there were 1.1 smokers per sign. For all of you using your fingers and toes as an abacus this equates to 22 smokers.

Hack, hack.

Now don't think that the PR consultants at Children's have gone Halliburton on us by charging money with no results. They have worked long nights by coming up with ingenious ideas intended solely to help out parents and visitors alike. For instance, the bathrooms are flooded with the scent of cinnamon. One would think that a fan would have been a good idea but apparently the over intoxicating aroma of an herb won out as the better solution. Don't look for this method to be adopted on any upcoming episodes of This Old House.

To combat feelings of depression the hospital has teamed up with concessions to provide a wide variety of healthy fruits and comfort foods like chips and chocolate. The chocolate is constantly sold out whereas the apples appear to be of plentiful supply!

If your waist line is further eroding your feelings of self esteem don't worry. The bathroom mirrors possess a convex appearance that makes everyone look somewhat taller and slimmer. This should help your general mood providing that you can stand the overpowering scent of cinnamon.

At least it covers up the second hand smoke still lingering on our clothes.

Brian & Deanna

Blog: Rigel 7

Submitted 10/03/2007

Body language tells us volumes about a person. For instance, it allows parents to get a jump start on knowing what the doctor is thinking. This knowledge helps us to formulate our next question or action and so forth. Keep in mind the deciphering body language is not an exact science. Sometimes we get it right and sometimes we don't. Actually, most times we don't. Can't blame us for trying though.

After all, we are part of the Start Trek generation. Ah yes, who can forget the lovable crew of Kirk, Spock, Bones and Scotty? How many episodes did we find the crew of the Enterprise stranded on a distant planet facing insurmountable odds? Even though, oddly enough, many of these aliens spoke perfect English it was up to Captain James T. Kirk to use his knowledge of body language to interpret his enemy's actions and save his crew.

Sure, a laser could have been used but Kirk preferred a different style. Shown in episodes 4, 8, 15, 27, 33, 42, 57 & 68 Kirk used this knowledge of alien body language to get his crew out of peril. Well, all except for the guys in the red shirts.

Less I digress.

Still, it is hard to make the leap of actions from Rigel 7 to the Children's PICU here on Earth. We all interpret human body language in different ways. In Zachary's case Deanna and I have to assemble this data from chatty doctors with stiff arms to monotone nurses with apparent seizure disorders. Some of the fellows are good communicators with bad eye contact while a few residents prefer to stare at their mobile computer screens and use email as their primary communication too.

Verbal discourse, body gestures or internet based answers...whatever works in this day and age. We may not be as good at it as Captain Kirk but then again, his show was canceled after three seasons.

Brian & Deanna

Blog: How Much?

Submitted 10/13/2007

How much would you pay in order to hold your child?

How big of a check would you write just to hear your spouse say "I love you"?

How much money would you, the reader, fork over just to see your best friend open their eyes and see your face?

Not my usual humorous or sarcastic beginning but they are good questions.

Deanna and I have not been able to hold Zachary for almost two months now. A beautiful baby caught in the middle of life's ugly tug-of-war. Even though he is laying in a crib, inches away from us, we can only touch him, talk to him and hope that he feels us holding his hand. A very rough stretch for a parent day in and day out.

Many people hold their kids and take that moment for granted. Trust me...it is a very precious point in time that is over way to fast.

We want to hold Zachary but can't. Perhaps tomorrow.

We want to cradle Zachary in our protective arms and shield from the evils of the world. Perhaps tomorrow.

It is unbearable to stare directly into Zac's closed eyelids and wonder if he knows that Mom & Dad are pulling for him. Well not tomorrow. This we experienced today!

Zachary's ICU doctors have been weaning him off of the narcotics over the past few days. The result is that our little trooper looks like he is coming out of a deep sleep and showing some general movements. Today both Deanna and I were watching over him as he open his eyes and looked right at us. A few seconds later Zac's sleepy *eyes soon drifted shut. The moment didn't last long. However, it was long enough!*

Brian & Deanna

Blog: Lost in Translation

Submitted 10/22/2007

It is important to know Zachary's condition in the present sense as well as the plan of attack for the next 24 hours. We get this information each and every morning when the doctors make their rounds. As a parent we get Gold Pass status which allows us to stand in the first class section with all of the white-lab-coat-wearing-medical-talking-clip-board-carrying-sky-high-student-loan-paying doctors. During rounds it can be very overwhelming listening to what amounts to a foreign language spit out at a high rate of speed. Consider listening to Stairway to Heaven from a 45 at 78.

What? Did I lose some of you? Google: "Record speed" or better yet, ask your parents.

As a responsible adult with a large assortment of 1980's power ties I feel that it is my duty to stand toe to toe with these MD folks. After all, I'm near average intelligence. I can get a few answers correct on the Jeopardy board. And yes, I feel that I'm smarter than a 5th grader. Surely the doctors can appreciate my hunger for medical knowledge and share ideas like colleges...or to a lesser degree, an irritating cousin at a family bbq.

Yet the group can be difficult to infiltrate. During rounds the doctors all huddle around each other like a football team announcing the next play. I feel like a spy or an outsider who is not really welcome but begrudgingly tolerated. The doctors review their notes so quietly that I have a hard time listening. Are they communicating telepathically? Special doctor sign language?

And in the end they all put their hands on top of each other, yell "Break" and come out with a plan of attack . The attending doctor always asks if we, the parents, have questions. After receiving their answers I wonder if there is something lost in translation between the attending doctor and the parents.
For instance, here is a brief clip of yesterday's rounds:

Doctor to staff: "Give Zac 65ml of 35% albumin, decrease his HCT from .75 to .5 and let's set him up on a Lasix drip with Ethacrynic Acid doses from Q12 to Q8. The x-rays look hazy too. Any questions?"

Brian's Thoughts: "Was that in English? Did I hear the word acid? Isn't acid bad? Quick, think of something intelligent sounding."
Brian: So, will this allow Zachary to get less puffy?

Doctor's Response: "Yes, this should be the best course of action for his weight and height."

Brian's Thoughts: "Puffy? Come on Johnson, you sound like an idiot. Everyone is watching. Ask a better question."
Brian: So, is 35% of albumin a low enough dose?
Brian's Thoughts: "Ah, good one. This will surely provoke some thoughtful response."

Doctor's Response: "This amount provides the best low volume intake. We could do 5% but this would add to his fluid overload. We want to stay away from that."

Brian Thoughts: "Ooooooookay, still not making any progress here. Change the topic! Point to the x-ray and deliver a commanding response."
Brian: So I've noticed the hazy part of the x-ray that you are referring to. This part is certainly clogged with moisture. How can we get this eliminated?"

Brian's Thoughts: *"Ah yes, an impressive question. One for the weekly highlights for sure. This shows my attention to detail and my understanding of the situation. Get prepared for the accolades."*

Doctor: *"Um, that white area that you are pointing to is his heart. We kinda need that."*

Brian's Thoughts: *"Is there a rock nearby that I can crawl under?"*

Brian & Deanna

Blog: Starbucks Factor

Submitted 10/11/2007

Actions associated with sights and sounds are a human trait. Since the days of cavemen and dinosaurs this connection is practically hardwired into our dna.

See mastodon.

Hear mastodon.

Throw rock at mastodon. Ug ug.

Fast forward few thousand years.

Lots of sights and sounds emanate from Zachary's bedside. This stands to reason I guess as there are lots of electrical gizmos surrounding his crib. From several pumps to a ventilator to a monitor there is always something going off telling the nurse to switch a vial, administer a drug or jiggle a line.

The other day one of theses alarms went off from one of Zachary's monitors. Physically I jumped out of my chair and tried to pinpoint the root of the problem. Ah, the third pump up from the bottom, second pole from the right. A red light is flashing! Mentally my brain raised the stress awareness level to Def Con 4. Surely Zachary's nurse and the entire squadron of medical folks would come walking...no, sprinting over to address this issue.

"Helloooooooooooooooooooooooooooooo".
"Bell ringing here".
"Red light flashing!"

Strangely enough, no one even raised an eye brow. Apparently my increased stress level was contained to me and me only. The entire staff continued their daily routines - no one even put down their coffee. Did I miss something here? Did my highly evolved caveman senses fail to grasp the true meaning of alarms and flashing red lights?

It dawned on me that my prehistoric mentality shouldn't be looking at such archaic and obvious signs. Forget the lights. Forget the alarms. No, the tall tale signs of emergency medical activity was based on a hot beverage. This is something that I will call: "The Starbucks Factor" which revolves around the following levels:

● **SBF 1** - Patient wakes up with a case of bad hair. Medical staff continues to order their lattes and cappuccinos through a nurse usually named Linda or Rick.
● **SBF 2** - Patient complains of ingrown toe nail. Medical staff may glance over at crib but continues to discuss who had the skinny mocha vs. whole milk.
● **SBF 3** - Patient develops a severe case of athlete's foot. Medical staff will walk over for a visual inspection but will never actually set their hot caffeinated beverage down. Usually they instruct Linda or Rick to rub ointment on affected areas.
● **SBF 4** - Patient's heart breaks out of chest cavity and rolls down hallway. Medical staff instantly throws empty latte containers in trash (half full lattes get set down gently on nearby shelf) and comes running. Usually Linda is knocked down in the process. Rick is instructed to go fetch runaway heart.

Like the mastodon of years past, the alarms and lights are at the end of their usefulness. Their time has come and gone.

> *Today's barometer of emergent activity is the coffee cup.*
>
> *Brian & Deanna*

Blog: Doctor Parent Bonding

Submitted 10/26/2007

As Zachary lies in bed in a sedated & paralyzed state we have ample opportunity to discuss his prognosis with the various ICU, Transplant or other doctors that seem to visit his bedside. Like sponges we try to absorb all of the various medical jargons that is used to describe why his condition improves or nose dives. Most of the explanations are one step above theory and are responded with polite nods or in my case, a hazy film developing over my eyes similar to what a deer sees when they look at the headlights of passing cars.

Usually at the end of this doctor-parent bonding sessions the doctor walks away with some sort of positive tort like "hang in there" or "lets keep our fingers crossed". The clichés are token at best and resembles some sort of opening dialogue from the bald-headed beat cop on Hill Street Blues. Of course all verbal quips are followed with some sort of hand gesture like a thumbs-up, crossed fingers or my favorite, the fist near the heart with the "soul man" double pump. Always a heart warming visual.

However, sometimes the doctor digs deep. I mean REALLY deep into their emotional bag of feelings and goes that extra step. Yes, I'm talking about that crater sized leap from hand gesture to physical touch. The kind of touch that is on par with a Hallmark card. The kind of touch that say they care the very best.

This type of action ranges from some sort of touch on the arm to a pat on the back. Ah yes, the rules certainly change when contact is involved. No longer is the dialogue meant as a passing comment with no expected reply.

Now, the doctor's comment is complimented with a lingering stare into the parent's pupils. As if to reinforce the warm & fuzzy nature of the touch the stare is done without a smile which makes it all the more awkward.

So what kind of response is expected here? Not entirely clear as this is certainly a case by case situation. However, the top choices are as follows:

1. Turn around and ask them to scratch that hard-to-reach spot in the middle of your back.
2. Copy the NFL players and give the doctor a pat on the bum when they walk away. Perhaps stating loudly something like "attaboy" or "attagirl".
3. Lean over and give the doctor a full body hug. Add to this some sort of soft spoken comment like "I've always admired you the most". Let the hug linger.

Personally I think the staff just feels guilty due to a lack of tv for Zac's crib!

Brian & Deanna

Blog: "The Intimidator" starring Deanna Johnson
Submitted 10/28/2007

A long time ago in a hospital far far away Zachary was born. During this initial stage of medical intervention we have had numerous conversations with the doctors and pretty much hung on their every word. After all, they knew the big words, had their own personal stethoscope around their necks and seemed to have some sort of bat phone connected to the Heavens!

We were newbies to this hospital flowchart. Visiting parents with no expiration date. From our point of view the hierarchy of medicinal care was an established and well running process. Who were we to question such a plan?

Doctors talk to God.
Nurses talk to the Saints.
Custodians talk to themselves.

There you have it. These simple rules are the basis for how instructions get carried out in a medical environment. These rules are essentially carved in granite. Like Moses' tablets, no one was going to question this process and risk being turned into salt. Okay, so I'm combining some biblical stories here but you get the point. But as we became more educated on the ways of Zac's health we tended to develop different views from the top down.

Last week Deanna threw the proverbial wrench into this time tested process. She actually questioned the doctor's thought process and suggested a different course of action for Zachary's health. GASP! For a split second the Earth stopped rotating. Seattle became sunny. The Cleveland Indians were winning. I even put my coffee cup down. What was happening to life as we know it?

To set things right a meeting between the doctor and "The Intimidator" was certainly needed. The deck of the USS Missouri seemed unlikely. Versailles was a tad far away. Fortunately a side room became available and Deanna was invited inside for the discussion. Like a principal asking the student into their office, Deanna entered the small room ready for battle. The doctor even asked one of the PICU patient's parents to leave the room so he could consult with his new adversary. "Let's close the door" he uttered. I'm sure that flashbacks of her troubled high school youth resurfaced.

In the end a brief conference was all that was needed for clarification. War had been averted. Zachary's care continued. No one turned into salt and Moses never turned over in his grave.

And I continued to drink my coffee.

Brian & Deanna

Blog: Scrubs

Submitted 11/28/2007

I was scanning the cable channels a few nights ago and came across one of those old black & white movies. I don't remember the name of the flick but it was set in a hospital surrounded with typical Hollywood props. There was the old cranky nurse, the twenty-something intern, the distinguished looking male doctor and of course the very sick yet very attractive looking patients. Apparently those doctors didn't have many diseases to cure back then but could always determine the cause of the sickness merely by shining a flashlight at the patient's pupils.

Most of the props that Hollywood had in place were comical by today's standards. The only part where they hit the bull's eye was attire. The doctors wore a shirt, tie and lab coat, the nurses wore white stockings, white shoes and the coup de grace, that white starchy hat. For comical relief there was always some sort of clerical person running around in a sweater vest. Clothing certainly helped the viewer identify who did what and thus helped us to understand the movie's plot.

Enter reality.

In today's hospital, employee attire is a little more on the confusing side. Figuring out who does what based upon clothing is about as easy as throwing a Yahztee. As parents of patients we take this opportunity to take on the role of a detective, hoping that clothing may give us clues as to what the employee does. Like in the movies today's doctors will from time to time wear nice clothing with their lab coats. But now they also routinely substitute scrubs under their lab coats or shed the coats entirely and just wear their scrubs.

Nurses are a tad more fashionable group it seems. They wear long sleeve shirts or some sort of nursing gown with little pictures of SpongeBob Squarepants or simply go casual and wear their scrubs. No matter what the attire, *one thing is for certain in today's PICU fashion show : no more white starchy hats.*

Let's not forget the respiratory people? They wear scrubs. Surgeons wear scrubs (both in and out of the OR). Physical therapy and occupational therapy all wear scrubs. So it seems as if everyone had begun their clothing inventory by shopping at Scrubs R Us. So does anyone new to the scene know who does what in a hospital setting? Not from my point of view.

In the end all I know is that no one in the hospital wears a sweater vest.

Brian & Deanna

Blog: Patience
Submitted 11/04/2007

During Zachary's 14 month hospital membership we have been inundated with information pertaining to medicinal care, insurance forms, and where to get free coffee. Throughout this ordeal there has been a tremendous give and take to our knowledge base. For instance, we have gained valuable insight on intestinal stuff like what part of the bowel absorbs nutrients vs. what part absorbs water. Great information for bar room trivia or perhaps when either Deanna or myself enter med school. The flip side though, is what aspect of our mental ability have we lost.

Could it be IQ points?
Reasoning ability?
Hair?
No to all of the above. The correct answer is Patience.

They say that patience is a virtue. Frankly, I believe that it is way over rated. The ability to restrain from urges like giving wedgies, noogies or asking questions that begin with "Are you out of your mind?" is just something that the human race has evolved to. Like the spleen, Deanna and I no longer have any use for this human virtue and routinely expect (if not demand) instant answers to our questions.

For example:

Deanna to Resident: "What plan do you have regarding Zachary's ventilator settings?"
Resident to Deanna: "Well..."

[Buzzer]

We feel that this question was not answered fast enough. My advice to the resident next time is to not use the term "Well... " with the optional dramatic pause. This implies that they don't know the answer and will probably subject us to some sort of theory. News Flash: We can theorize. We don't want theories. We want facts. Stat.

You can't really blame us for the drop in patience. After all, everyone is picking up the pace in life. For example, when one is hungry and fast food isn't quick enough, we do the drive-thru. Cash taking too long? Use plastic! Anything under $20 doesn't require a signature. I mean who wants to wait around an extra 10 seconds to sign a sales slip? Who has that kinda time?

Thus patience seems to be a passing fad like poodle skirts, 8-tracks and those incredibly ugly horned rimmed glasses that I see in all of my brother's high school senior album pictures. What were those people thinking back in 1976?

Of course, the reality of the situation is that Zachary is taking his time on the healing front and couldn't care less about schedules. It is amazing that a 14 month old can teach such lessons in humility to adults without uttering a single word.

Amazing indeed.

Brian & Deanna

Blog: Groundhog Day

Submitted 11/08/2007

It seems like the past few months Deanna and my life are similar to the movie Groundhog Day. Each day we wake up by our alarm clock (which incidentally sounds a lot like Aidan waking up), grab a quick shower, breakfast and the day is officially under way. One of us arrives at the hospital to catch the early morning rounds with Zachary's medical staff while the other stays at home with Aidan. At lunch time we switch. The next day is pretty much an exact repeat.

Thus the days are blending into one. The weeks are indistinguishable. The name of the current month is a blur. Simply replace the town of Punxsutawney with Pittsburgh and the word sequel comes to mind. Groundhog Day 2: The Search for Sanity.

While we wait for a movie company to buy the rights to this story we continue to adapt to our new lives in the Steel City. It's been awhile since either of us has lived in an apartment. In a way I feel like we have gone back in time to our college days. In addition to the compacted way of living, we have a limited budget. We sit on donated furniture. We take the bus. There is more macaroni and cheese in our cabinets and grocery coupons are not automatically thrown out but filed for future trips to the market.

Don't get me wrong, **<sarcasm on>** apartment life isn't all fun and games **<sarcasm off>**. There are some obvious drawbacks to this lifestyle. For instance, having neighbors living so close that they can hear your shower turn on isn't exactly comforting. Finding a parking spot on the street proves to be more demanding than finding weapons of mass destruction.

And when tomorrow comes we get to do it all over again.

Brian & Deanna

Blog: Half Full
Submitted 11/25/2007

As parents we try to have an optimistic view on Zachary's condition...or at least we try to lean in that direction. We are the "glass is half full" kinda people. Living in the present yet looking forward with hope is the PICU religion we adhere to. Thinking any different is just not in the cards.

On Saturday Zachary looked great. Better than great. He was off of the BiPap machine, awake, smiling with all of his four teeth and giving all around him a huge dose of the warm & fuzzies. The hard part seemed a distant past, buried in some lost quadrant of our brain's memory cells. It was time to discuss Zac's exodus plan from the PICU. It was time to discuss possible discharge. It was time to discuss little league, junior high school and the prom.

We left the PICU on Saturday night with high hopes. This was certainly a cause for celebration as the wine glasses were more than half full that evening. However, early Sunday morning the other shoe dropped. An infection was detected: gram negative rods. Nasty bug. Damn!

Zachary did an admiral job of fighting this bacteria for awhile but at around midnight he began to struggle a bit. The decision was made to help him out and put him back on the ventilator. Yes, the dreaded machine that we have formed a love-hate relationship with was once again sitting beside our son's bed.

We are once again reminded of just why we are in Pittsburgh. It is time to discuss the present with the PICU

docs. It is time to formulate a game plan for Zac's recovery. Little league can wait. For now that is.
   After all, the glass is half full.

Brian & Deanna

Blog: Eye Contact

Submitted 11/30/2007

   During my college years I held many jobs. One in particular was a seasonal holiday position at a Lima, Ohio department store. My job was to service the floor that overlooked both toys and guns. Yes, you read correctly. I was essentially paid to keep Cabbage Patch Dolls and Winchester 12 gauge shotguns fully stocked on neighboring shelves. Apparently someone at the home office thought that these two areas of products had some sort of distant relationship. Perhaps 5th cousin, 4th at best.

   So during the holiday shopping rush it was routine for some frantic parent to track me down, inform me that the shelf was empty and politely order me to go searching for little Sally's favorite toy back in the warehouse. Upon my return there was yet another frantic parent holding on to their version of Santa's list. Back to the warehouse I went...and again and again and again.

   In order to do my job and keep the shelves stocked I quickly learned two valuable lessons:
1. Don't linger on the shopping floor.
2. Never make eye contact with parents.

   Here at the PICU there is a similar scenario. This time the stock boys are the various doctors from the Transplant team. Their job is to help locate the organ equivalent of Barbie's Malibu collection. The frantic parents are, well, they are people like Deanna and me. It is our job to track them down and inquiry in 30 words or less how things are going.

I've noticed that these doctors have learned the same valuable lessons. Like my minimum wage job, they tend not to hang out in the PICU. And when they do they typically don't make eye contact with folks like me. When necessary they come in the room for a quick consult and exit the nearest door. Quick, efficient and stealthy, these docs have intimate knowledge of the floors blueprints which help them to avoid the likes of me.

So in the meantime Deanna and I sit by Zachary's crib and focus on the positive stuff. We talk about his improved vital signs, strong heartbeat and the bad haircut that our nurse received. Sometimes we see the transplant doc and in the blink of an eye they are gone. Must have been a hidden trap door.

We need to get copies of those blueprints.

Brian & Deanna

Blog: Third Time's a Charm
Submitted 12/07/2007

As I stepped out of my apartment building this morning I was pelted in the face by Old Man Winter's arsenal of snow flakes. During my short walk from building door to bus stop I was morphed from my usual GQish looking fashionable ensemble to that of a snow man in hand me downs from K-Mart.

Oh yeah, December – must be winter.

Time to bundle up, break out the parkas and forget about hair style. Winter is a time for heavy sweaters, bad hair and the eventual wait for the warmth of spring. Waiting, however is not Zachary's style. This past week has shown tremendous improvement is all areas. Let me catch everyone up on the progress.

First of all Zachary was extubated last week. I have put off announcing this big news primarily for superstitious reasons. You see the last two times I made such fan fare on extubation Zachary was soon put back on the ventilator. Perhaps I jinxed it. However, as the saying goes: third time's a charm. So here we are.

Secondly, the infection that Zac caught has been successfully fought off. Thanks in part to his improved condition as well as rapidly dispensed antibiotics. His condition has improved so much that he has been moved from the PICU on the 6th floor to a step down unit up on the 7th floor.

This move possesses some mixed blessings:

Good Points:
- *Private Room.*
- *TV (sorry, no HBO).*
- *Our very own bathroom.*
- *View of an a/c unit through window. Don't laugh too much, as far as air conditioners go, this is a nice one.*

Bad Points:
- *Nursing ratio changes from 1:1 to 2:1 or even 3:1.*
- *Have to learn nurse's names all over again.*
- *Lost is the entertainment value of watching staff in PICU.*
- *One more flight of stairs to walk up.*

The most dramatic change this past week is our ability to hold Zachary. Without the breathing tubes limiting his mobility we can now scoop up his little frame to hold him, squeeze him and call him George (anyone remember this Bugs Bunny skit?).

Wait! There's more! We have seen more smiles and giggles from Zachary this past week than we have EVER seen. He loves his toys and utters some sort of noise whenever we put them in his crib. Remember that he did have a tube in his throat for three months so screaming is a tad hard to do. Give him some time. In the meantime we wait for him to say our names with some sort of British accent like Tiny Tim in A Christmas Carol. "Muhther, Fahther, may I 'ave a spot of tea in my bottle?"

Keep in mind that he will still need the organ transplants. No getting around this hard core fact. But the progress that he has made since his life flight from Johns Hopkins more than three months ago is amazing. Waiting for improvement is over. Spring has arrived in Zac's room.

Dad's bad hair...well I'll work on that.

Brian & Deanna

Blog: *Trending North*

Submitted 12/09/2007

So now that Zachary's health appears to be positive and trending north we are now faced with a whole new set of issues to deal with. As he gets better and better Zac is subject to yet another possible move by Children's U-Haul department to another step down unit.

"Ah, this sounds great" you say.

"Oh contraire" I reply in my best French sounding accent.

If Zachary moves to a step down unit then his points on the transplant list also move down. Less points means less urgent status on the list. This equates to organs going to another deserving child. Which in turn means more wait time for us. Zac's future is becoming complicated and requires some thought.

So, placement on "The List" is everything. "The List" is sorta all encompassing like "The Force" for Star Wars fans. Every night we hope that the phone will ring from the Transplant doc telling us that a donor has been found. Can't visualize? How about Luke Skywalker telling R2D2 *that he found a new computer chip for his ailing operating system? Imagine how thrilled C3PO would be knowing that his android friend would be around for the sequel.*

Why do I always get on these sci fi tangents?

So currently Zachary is chilling in his private room with the garden view of an HVAC machine on the step down unit on the 7th floor. When the doctors come in to inquire about Zachary I feel that we are cast into the role of our son's coach relaying sporting information to the press. When the doctors ask us how Zachary is doing I find myself in an odd position. Do I smile and say "He's doing good Doc" or do I lie and say "He's not doing good Doc. He has clammy hands and can't form cohesive sentences".

Like the BCS we have no idea of the future and are trying to take this situation one day at a time. What I do know is that each and every day Deanna and I hold Zachary and marvel at how many teeth are forming in his mouth. We are happy that his hair is growing. We get a kick out of hearing him giggle, laugh and smile.

Perhaps thinking of the future isn't as important as living in the present.

Brian & Deanna

Blog: Reality Programs

Submitted 12/16/2007

Not so long ago there was time when Deanna and I would spend our Seattle nights curled up in front of the fireplace – our bellies full from dinner and getting ready to see what cable television had in store for our entertainment that evening. Life was slower paced back then. Responsibilities were at a minimum. Our border collie Bailey snoozed on the couch and had our undivided attention. What to watch that night? Comedy? Drama? Reality?

Our lives have certainly taken a different path since then. Unless you are new to this site and haven't read the prior 54 posts (go ahead, we'll wait) you know that Deanna and I have moved to Maryland just in time to unpack and now temporarily relocate to the snow belt of Pittsburgh. No longer do we view Mt. Rainier but now look out at the Pitt's Cathedral of Learning. No longer do we kayak Chesapeake Bay but commute to the hospital on the #500 bus.

Welcome to Transplant Central.

Each week there is a new attending doctor who's job is to monitor their patients and make them better. At the end of the week they pass the baton to another attending doctor who is, essentially the next person on the medical relay time. Sometimes Zachary has a good week and sometimes he doesn't. Consequently we favor the doctors during the good weeks and frown upon the others. My suggestion here is to borrow from the script of Survivor and vote one of the doctors out of the PICU. Not permanently mind you but for a few months or so. Maybe bring them back for a guest appearance during Sweeps Week.

Perhaps there are other areas of hospital situations that could be improved upon. Could it be that I'm on to something here? Maybe my endless hours of watching NBC, ESPN and HBO could be an asset. Perhaps there are other reality programs that we can borrow from:

Extreme Makeover: *How about we get the skinny guy with the funny goatee to round up a few hundred volunteers with hammers and tool belts and build us PICU parents a new state of the art waiting room. Equipped with big screen gas plasma tv, mini bar and artificial turf with huge recliners set around the 50 yard line. "Busdriver, move that crib".*

Biggest Loser: Since Zachary has ballooned up a few times only to lose the water weight over a few weeks it makes sense to reward him for this weight loss. Bring in the personal trainers (I think they are called physical therapists) and enter him in the competition. I'll admit that we have a slight edge in this contest as Deanna is a pediatric physical therapist herself. Keep that secret between us.

What Not to Wear: It seems that Zachary is always wearing the same Pampers #3 diaper. How lame is that? Perhaps we locate a fashion guru to come in and suggest other brands, other colors or sizes. How about a braided belt or red suspenders. Maybe get some alternative clothing for the staff as opposed to scrubs. Personally I'd like to see more hiking boots, flannel lab coats and the optional Birkenstocks sandals.

The Apprentice: This could be something tailored only for the new staff of the PICU. It would be their job to work long hours, go without sleep and ask to do all of the chores that no one else has time for. Oh wait, they are already doing this. They are called Residents.

The Amazing Race: Parents of patients have to compete in teams against time and unseemly in achievable goals. For instance the parents have to find anyone at the Financial Aid office (who is always on a lunch break), then locate a copier (I have yet to find one) and finally find a parking place after 12pm. Good luck.

As television evolves backwards in quality programming it may be wise to consider other options. A good book. A glass of wine or a family of four. Off the couch Bailey, make room for Aidan and Zachary.

Brian & Deanna

Blog: *Crusin' 7 North*

Submitted 12/19/2007

Yesterday Zachary was relocated to another step down unit called 7 North. This ward, just down the hall from his previous home at 7 South is pretty much for pre and post transplant patients. The reason for the move is simple enough. He is getting better.

Define better please?

Well, for starters he has been off of the ventilator and other types of breathing assistance for a few weeks now. He is also off of the medications that helped with his blood pressure and many of his electrolytes are stable. He is able to sit up and play with toys and read fine literature like Brown Bear Brown Bear and The Adventures of Pooh.

Probably the most important part is that Deanna and I can walk around the ward with Zac and give him a view of something other than his room. Kinda like crusin' the 7 North strip. A lot of cute babies to babble with.

Consider this visual: Deanna and I hold Zac with one arm and pull his various supporting pumps with the other. We may not be in the best cardio shape but our arms are bulking up.

Zachary is currently on a plan to get weaned off of the pain medications. Apparently our son developed quite a liking for these drugs during his four month (and counting) stay. This is quite normal they say as his dealer...I mean his doctor is now trying to back down slowly to avoid withdrawals. As I reach for my much needed daily pot of coffee I wonder just how someone can get addicted to this type of medication.

Even though Zachary is showing great strides of improvement keep in mind that there is no evidence that his liver and small bowel are getting better. Yeah, it would be a nice Christmas present but the likelihood of this happening is about as probable as a toxic bite from a *spider giving me the ability to shoot strands of silk from my wrists.*

So in the meantime we wait for organs...and cruise 7 North looking for chicks!

Brian & Deanna

Blog: A Good Night's Sleep

Submitted 12/23/2007

When I was around 5 years of age I contacted bronchitis and had to spend a fair amount of time in the local hospital. I don't remember much about the medical side of my stay but I do remember that the nurses insisted on keeping the door of my room open. An open door policy may have been convenient for their job but it played havoc with my sleep schedule.

First of all there was a bright light in the hallway whose secondary function was to shine it's 200 watt light rays directly into my eye sockets. With fused retinas and a rapidly forming tan line on my face any chance of sleep was soon diminished. Add to this optical impairment a healthy dose of constant interruptions from the nursing staff and I was destined to be a cranky patient.

A good night's sleep was never had.

That was over thirty years ago and I wonder just how far we have come in the medical establishment. Oh sure today's staff is probably better trained, the equipment is far superior and the student loans are higher. But based on recent experiences I am not exactly inspired with confidence that today's patients get a higher dose of quality sleep.

To throw some up front compliments here let me state that Zachary's room is a nice size. It has a private bath, a window and some very talented and nurturing nurses. The doctors seem to be on top of his every move and always make time to answer our questions and discuss our concerns. However, everyone agrees that in order for Zachary to get better, he needs his rest.

Here is where the irony begins.

In order for Zachary to sleep he needs something called silence - a rare commodity at 7 North. The reasons are pretty straightforward actually. For one, the helicopter pad is located pretty close to Zac's window. I can feel the vibrations as the fan blades resonate through his window [wump] [wump] [wump]. There are a handful of bells that go off whenever his blood pressure, heart rate or breathing approaches a set number [beep] [beep] [beep]. There are alarms that sound when his medication pump finishes up on delivering the proper dosage of drugs [ding] [ding] [ding]. Did I mention that there is an intercom located three feet from his crib [yakety] [yakety] [yakety]?

Granted, he is in the hospital and alarms are meant to be loud and irritating. Staff has to enter the room in order to do their jobs. Intercoms are necessary for good communication. All of this I understand! Still even though Zac is nestled all snug in his bed, it makes it hard for him to dream of sugar plums dancing in his head.

Perhaps Zachary doesn't need more sedation drugs but something old school like a good pair of ear plugs.

Brian & Deanna

Blog: Sometimes Y

Submitted 1/03/2008

Confusion starts early in one's life. Consider a rite of passage. A requirement into adulthood if you will. Personally I think that it started with the whole Santa Claus thing. I mean, as a kid there was no fireplace in our house. How did the fat jolly guy enter our dwelling?

In elementary school we were taught how to spell with so many caveats that it is amazing that anyone can spell at all. Remember I Before E except after C? How does one explain words like seizure, heist or weight? Good thing that the letter C is not in those words. My, that would really get confusing. Then how do we explain society?

Remember A E I O U and sometimes Y? When Y? Sometimes. Sometimes? Well, not all the time...just sometimes. **<sarcasm on>** Oh, that makes sense **<sarcasm off>.** Can't wait for the spelling test.

Confusion certainly is a staple food item in our nutritional makeup of education.

When Deanna asked the doctors a few weeks back about the possibility Zachary's discharge we were given somewhat vague and ambiguous answers. One doctor favors this week for various reasons while another favors next week for different reasons. One doctor thought that we had to wait until Zachary got a little more healthy but failed to define what healthy was. Three doctors, three different answers.

Sometimes Y.

Last week Zachary was taken off all of the sedation drugs. Well, lately we've noticed that he is starting to exhibit signs of withdrawal. Not a lot of obvious signs mind you but enough to know that something was off a tad. This necessitated the reintroduction of the sedative Methadone. When will this be weaned off? I'm told a few days or a week. Could be more. Hard to answer really.

Sometimes Y.

Since many aspects of Zachary's health changes from one day to the next, pinning the docs down on issues like discharge date is like hitting a moving target. I'm not really blaming the medical staff for the wide net of vague answers (okay, maybe a little), I just want them to reign it in some.

Part of the problem is that each doctor seems to be reading a different version of the same text book. Is it possible to get all of these folks on the same page?

Perhaps we can get our border collie Bailey to herd them all into one room so we can get a group consensus on what to expect and go from there.

Then we can finally define Sometimes Y.

Brian & Deanna

Blog: Mr. Johnson

Submitted 1/29/2008

Parent's names are an immaterial piece of information within Children's Hospital walls. Even though we all have them plastered on our credit cards, driver's license or Blockbuster video card there seems to be no need for them at this venue. As parents we are simply known as "Mom" or "Dad". Simply. Quick. Easy.

The reasons for this are muddled in some obscure form of hospital-parent logic. It seems that as parents we pretty much lose all type of identity the moment we enter the front door. We are sorta like the less attractive friend on a double date. Oh sure, the nurse greets us and even asks how we are doing but they really don't care. After all, it is not us that they are taking care of. Their greeting to us is more of a token of formality. The main attraction here is Zachary. No offense taken - we're on board with this.

Imagine my confusion the other day when one of the Resident doctors called me Brian.

Brian?

Well, it's not like I've never heard this name before. After all, it is on my birth certificate. It is the name that people have been calling me since the LBJ Administration – the first one. If necessary I can further consult with my parents on this but I'm pretty sure that I have no other aliases.

So why did this name make me turn my head?

It seems that the unwritten rules of names are at the discretion of the doctors. The older Attending doctors seem to prefer a more formal approach and tend to call me Mr. Johnson. To be honest I'm not especially keen on this term. I'm too young to be called Mr. Johnson.

After all, I'm part of the high speed internet generation. I use text messaging. I shop at the Gap. When I hear Mr. Johnson I fully expect to see my dad standing behind me (who incidentally doesn't text message or shop at the Gap). These are the kind of doctors who flat out refuse to wear scrubs without at least a tie underneath.

Then there are the Fellows. This is the class of doctors who spent their college years watching reruns of Seinfeld. Like the majority of staff at Children's they prefer the term "Mom" or "Dad". They appear to be a little more relaxed in their appearance preferring Reeboks or Crocs (plastic garden shoes) with their attire. Sometimes they wear scrubs and sometimes their clothing suggests that they are heading out to Applebee's after rounds.

Let's not forget the Residents. This segment of doctors spends their free time discussing cool cell phones, Macs or favorite cast members from Dawson's Creek. This group is a little different as they don't introduce themselves with the surname "doctor" but prefer their first names like Devin or Cassie. The doctor part is simply implied and as one resident pointed out to me last week that it is also embroidered on his lab coat. Hmm, hard to argue with that logic.

I'm not saying that these people are more casual than others but I wouldn't be surprised if they came rolling up to Zachary's crib on a skateboard jamming to Green Day on their IPod.

All these doctors have their own style and hands down are exceptionally very smart and have kept Zachary in the running for organs. So who cares what they call me.

Just don't call me Mr. Johnson.

Brian & Deanna

Blog: *Time To Reboot*

Submitted 1/12/2008

The pendulum continues to swing in Zachary's favor as his overall health shows improvement. He is more energetic and continues to transition from less hours of sleep to more hours of play. The medications continue to decline and he is showing more enthusiasm with toys, books and cartoons as well as the desire to take the usual mid day nap.

So as Zac's Health Based Tilt O' Meter continues to point towards the positive side we see the reality of the inevitable discharge in the not to distant future. When in the future? Well, not too far into the future. We were hoping for a few days. A week maybe. February perhaps.

Why the uncertainty? It seems that Maryland Medicaid continues to confuse us for their requirements for payments. This process is about as easy to figure out as a Rubik's Cube. To combat these endless amounts of hurdles we have composed our own triangular team of problem solvers. From Deanna and myself to the staff at Children's to the folks from Johns Hopkins we have been manning the phones like political pollsters trying to get to the bottom of the issue.

Unfortunately it's a very deep hole.

It sounds great that so many people are trying to make this work but in the meantime the Johnson clan still has to make preparations for the future. So even though we know that Zachary will be discharged, the problem is that we were not exactly sure just where he would be discharged to.

As a pawn of the insurance game we had begun making parallel plans from both our apartment in Pittsburgh as well as our home in Severna Park. Trying to figure out this multi-platform configuration is like relearning algebra. Ouch, our brains are reaching their limits of capacity. Like our Windows based computer, we were unable to process any more data.

In the meantime we walk around our apartment, the hospital, even this city in what could be described as a constant state of confusion. Like zombies from a 1950's horror film we shuffle our feet and utter some small words as we make it through the day. Somehow we make it back and forth from apartment to hospital hoping not to be picked up by the psych ward – mistaken for lost patients.

Time to reboot.

Brian & Deanna

Blog: CNN

Submitted 1/15/2008

You can tell right away when it is a slow news day. The CNN anchor leads in with stories of cute puppies, the price of gasoline and how yet another singer/actor checked into rehab. Sometimes we watch the program and even find some pleasure in knowing that if this is the worst that the newscaster has to offer then maybe this isn't such a bad day after all. After all, no bad news is good news. Or so the saying goes.

Same thing on the Zachary front as there is nothing really new to report. We are still in limbo waiting for a decision to be made on the discharge. Lately I feel like I'm an investigative reporter asking the hard questions to some of the doctors in charge of this kind of thing. To be fair to them, this is not the norm in this wide wide world of discharge. They are essentially coordinating Zac's care with another facility, another pharmacy, another set of eyes. It takes some time as everyone involved has to be on the same page.

Barring any major issues, the latest and greatest is that Zachary will be discharged in a few days. We will probably transport him via our Honda CR-V with my John Denver collection playing the entire way. Now that I think of it, even I'm not sure that I can listen to Denver for 4 ½ hours. Still, we plan on leaving with a full tank of gas, a clean windshield and a few bags of greasy Doritos helping us to navigate the Pennsylvania Turnpike.

After we arrive at our Severna Park house I anticipate doing whatever stuff a family does when they arrive back at home after being in a hospital for the past four months. In other words, we'll wing it. "Winging it", by definition will probably involve getting the fridge restocked, testing the furnace and the reconnection of internet services. Somewhere in this mix a pot of coffee will be brewed and injected directly into my veins.

Soon afterwards, we will have to hook up with the Johns Hopkins GI team and let them get reacquainted with Zachary. Then we get to resume a somewhat normal lifestyle until we get a call for organs.   That alone should make for an interesting day.

Maybe CNN could lead in with that.

Brian & Deanna

Blog: Whack A Mole

Submitted 1/29/2008

Remember going to the arcade hall and playing your favorite games? There was pinball, ski ball, Pac man, air hockey and other various noisy machines. I wasn't especially good at any of these games but since it only took a quarter it was still fun to play. Now, of course some of the new games cost a small fortune to play and usually take dollars, Visa or gold bullion. The innocence of fun certainly comes with a price.

But then again, my wallet prefers the older games. Remember Whack-A-Mole?   This game required the skill to pound plastic gophers (well, they looked like gophers) with a mallet as they popped out of holes at quick random intervals. The faster you whacked the faster the varmints popped up. As the game progressed it became harder and harder to whack these little figurines.

Zachary's case is a little like this arcade game. The gophers are the various electrolytes that seem to pop up and throw his system in a state of turmoil. As soon as the doctors take care of a low electrolyte then another pops up. This series of problems, it seems, never ends.

Last week the problem was calcium. Normal levels of this mineral usually range from 8.5 to 10.5. Usually Zachary is right on target but for some reason he was registering something around 13. After playing with his intravenous fluids the docs finally got this electrolyte into the proper range.

Whack Whack

This week the culprits were potassium, sodium, ammonia, withdrawal and sedation issues. Again, the docs tweaked the fluids and added some supplements in order to balance out most of these areas. Of course each time something goes out of normal range we as parents get stressed. We have learned from experience that as something goes wrong it is because of something else.

It's the something else that scares us.

It seems as if something else arrived today. Step back to yesterday afternoon to where Zachary was having some problems settling down. After his scheduled dose of sedation we noticed that something just wasn't jiving as he was still somewhat agitated and breathing in light short breaths. These are not really the signs of a fully rested and relaxed child. What was going on?

Early this morning we got word from the doctors that Zachary's breathing was compromised and again back in the PICU on the ventilator. Every time this has happened in the past five months (I've lost track of the exact count) we were surprised and shocked. This time we kinda saw it coming.

So here is what we know: In spite of the ventilator, Zachary is still having some issues with his breathing. Add to this situation a newly developed fever, high ammonia amounts, concerns with lung x-rays and the usual liver related problems. The doctors certainly have their work cut out for them this week.

Whack Whack, Whack Whack

Still we are optimistic that Zachary will fight back these setbacks with some sort of incredible inner strength that amazes his nurses, his family and of course his parents. So tomorrow we will hang out by his crib and watch his doctors play Whack-A-Mole with his issues.

Deanna and I will provide the quarters.

Brian & Deanna

Blog: Facial Expressions

Submitted 2/15/2008

There are many times that I marvel at the way doctors handle the meetings with parents. There is no doublt that they have a very difficult job in conveying the patient's *condition in a straightforward articulate manner. Oh sure, the doctors have gone through 8 years of medical school to become well versed in the academics of medicine. They have done a lifetime of internships, residencies and fellowships that allow them to do their jobs with precision. Add to this verbal exchange the fact that the news is not always good news.*

Yet they always seem to keep the human element in the mix and accompany their information exchange with the appropriate FE (Facial Expression). It's like watching the 6 o'clock news where the anchor reports on drive by shootings (serious look), tax rates (concerned look) and spelling bee winners (happy look) with a seamless transition.

The doctors usually lead off the conversation with an overview of the current situation followed by their prognosis. Although no punches are pulled the doctors do in fact try to emphasis the positive points during their discussions. These positive points are their transition into the last portion of the conversation which hopefully ends on an upbeat note.

Here is an example of today's afternoon rounds:

Doctor: *Zachary's ammonia level is up again; his bilirubin continues to increase as well as his liver clotting factors. His potassium is low so we have to continue to give him syringes of this element. We feel that he has a little too much water in him so we will keep giving him the diuretic drip.* **FE**: *Frown*

Doctor: *Zachary's ammonia level is still drifting up at parts of the day. We are not sure of the reason and want to monitor this several times a day. We will increase his Lactulose and hope that this helps to correct the situation. We just can't figure our why it is so inconsistent.* **FE**: *Furrowed brow*

Doctor: Since his blood cultures have not grown anything we can assume that he is not infected with anything viral or bacterial. So we will discontinue the antibiotics Vancomycin and Meropenem. Since we are still concerned that this may resurface we will continue to monitor his temperature and blood pressures just in case. *FE*: Raised eyebrow

Doctor: With his net fluid intake we are hopeful that he will not need anymore diuretics after today. Perhaps we will stop this later this evening. This should help keep his potassium levels consistent. That should be one more pump we can put away in storage. *FE*: Smirk

Doctor: There is some good news here. Zachary's ventilator settings are being weaned down to a very low level. Barring anything negative in the next 24 hours it looks as if we will be removing the ventilator by tomorrow afternoon. *FE:* Smile

I look forward to when both Deanna and I can hold Zachary and walk around the step down unit at 7 North. Perhaps watching some cartoons or ESPN.
Just not the 6 o'clock news.

Brian and Deanna

Blog: *Pair Of Threes*

Submitted 2/20/2008

As we straddle the fence between parental hope and mental breakdown we have ample time to sit back and wonder about it all. Why are we in this situation? Why did Zachary get the short end of the stick? Why us? Of course there is no rationale to this equation but rather just the cards that life has dealt us. Not a very good hand I'll admit. It is like a pair of threes. Not much to bluff on.

But I suppose that child hurdles are something all parents experience. It's how you deal with them that defines your ratings as a parent. Even as the mountain of problems appears insurmountable we cannot simply call time out and take a vacation. I wish that it were that simple. So as Zachary's health changes from one day to the next we have to adjust our state of mind and deal with the situation at hand. In this arena of uncertainly it is our continuing job to simply be there for our son.

Of course this is a parent's job. It's our number one priority. During this entire hospital stay we realize that complaining doesn't help. Wishing for something won't make it happen. Knowing the facts may help us to communicate with the doctors but in the end it is like reading tea leaves. There is no better fast track to Stressville than the feeling of helplessness.

And let's be clear here – at times there can be a tremendous amount of stress.

Zachary's daily labs are not very promising. His respiratory system is shaky. His immune system is showing signs of deterioration. Most importantly, his liver is on borrowed time as it is. The physical part we have some experience in dealing with. The mental aspect is another story.

I'm sure Zachary doesn't appreciate the noise, the lights and the constant interruptions while lying in his crib. I imagine that he wonders just why he has to stay in his room while Aidan gets to go home with Mom and Dad. And I'm sure that he is not very happy with all of these wires and tubes attached to his body. Yet this is the way that it is.

As parents it is very humbling to accept this fact. Worse yet is that you just can't do anything about it. In the end all we can do is hold him and love him until things get better.

I hope this it is enough.

Brian & Deanna

Blog: Trial Run

Submitted 2/23/2008

We all strive for consistency in our lives. It's what gets us through the day with the least amount of stress. This doesn't mean that we are boring folks. Not at all. We can appreciate a little spontaneity like the next person... just as long as we can properly plan and prepare for it.

I guess this is why Zachary's situation is so hard to deal with. After all, he doesn't wait until after 5pm for his blood tests to throw a jolt of scare into us. He doesn't wait for weekends or any other convenient time to bump up the stress level. He just doesn't seem to want to play by the rules.

Could this be the tall tell signs of the beginning of a troublemaker?

A rebel without a cause?

On Wednesday evening we received a phone call from one of the doctors on the transplant team. Apparently an organ donor was found for Zachary in Georgia. It was all preliminary of course but there were many good signs to justify proceeding forward. Although we were given limited information we knew that the donor was a five day old newborn. His blood type was "O" which is compatible with Zachary's "A+".

The doctor stated a few times that nothing was for sure and that the chance of transplant was still 50-50. Of course this is not how my brain interpreted his statements. I heard something like "Congratulations. All of your problems will be gone by tomorrow".

By the morning the nursing staff had transported Zachary from 7 North to the O.R to begin prepping for surgery. Even though you want to hold off on the good news until you are absolutely sure it is a go you can't help but start the internal celebration. I must admit that I was starting to feel pretty optimistic. After all this time Zachary was finally going to get his transplant. My dream of playing catch with the twins in the back yard was becoming a little clearer.

Then we got the word that there will be no transplant. The organs, as it turns out, were not up to the strict levels demanded by the transplant team. From what they tell us, the intestines didn't pass the preliminary tests. Bottom line: bad stock.

Stop the prepping.

End the optimism.

Return back to Earth.

Even though the previous sleepness night yielded nothing, we feel encouraged that Zachary was considered for transplant. We learned that he is not only at the top of the transplant list in the Pittsburgh region but in the entire country as well. So we wait a few more days (weeks or months) for the next call. Consider this a trial run.

In the meantime I will discuss with Zachary the rules of life. After all, no one wants a troublemaker.

Brian & Deanna

Blog: Persona Upgrade

Submitted 3/02/2008

No matter what subject in life you discuss there is always that one person who has to one up you. You know these people. They always have more stress than you. They have more aches and pains than you. Their kids are stronger, faster and smarter than yours.

I remember when Deanna and I reached our five year anniversary there was a lady who had to undermine this occasion by telling us that we had to be married for 20 years to get a true perspective on the subject. Now that we have kids there was a guy who informed us that we really needed to wait until the junior high years to appreciate how stressful life can be. It seems that the initiation ritual into the University of Bragging Rights is never ending.

It's a good thing that I am above all of that.

But lately I may be falling from my perch. Perhaps now that the shoe is on the other foot I have more in common with these folks than I care to admit. It seems that my persona has been upgraded to Brian 2.0.

Since Deanna and I are hospital bound pretty much all day long it is really difficult to discuss world affairs with Zachary or his other 2 year old friends. So as I routinely strike up conversations with other parents of patients at 7 North, the topic of "Why are you here?" inevitably comes up. It seems a normal subject. After all, we aren't here for vacation reasons.

The other day I was talking to a dad who told me that his daughter has been here a whole week. "A whole week" I thought to myself, "wait until you have been here a few months". Just yesterday I was discussing transplant stuff with a parent of a little boy. His dad told me that he needed a heart. "Just one organ" I thought to myself. "Wait until you need a few more".

It appears that I am officially turning into those other people. Of course it is only a matter of time until I actually say out loud what I've been thinking. Once the dam has burst it will soon be common for me to discuss things like 8-tracks, party lines and how life was before microwaves, ATMs and remote controls.

Looks like I don't have to wait until the junior high years after all.

Brian & Deanna

Blog: A Good Closing

Submitted 3/07/2008

Bedside manor is a very important trait among all people in the medical community. Some people exude this ability in mass while others...well, let's just say that they fall somewhat short. However, no matter how good or bad the bedside rhetoric it can always be salvaged or destroyed by the last sentence. A good closing is a must in all doctor patient communications.

But like all good closings there is always something extra in the mix. A smile, for example done correctly will bridge the gap between a so-so meeting and a positive ending. A nod of the head with raised eyebrows works in a pinch. But the granddaddy of them all is some sort of physical touch.

Touching the parents is by all accounts an art form. Done right, the effect can bring comfort to a very stressful situation. It's a type of connection with the parent that, when appropriate, allows the doctors to ratchet it up a few notches and show their human side. Keep in mind that it's not for everyone as not all doctors adhere to the Reach Out and Touch Someone policy.

For those who prescribe to an Open Touch policy, there are many types of examples to choose from regardless of gender, age or even experience. With several months of note taking compiled while at Children's I feel like I have accumulated a wealth of statistical data on the subject. Perhaps there is enough for a good episode on Dateline or at the very least, a small black & white pamphlet at the local free clinic.

The following are the various kinds of touch broken down in paragraph form:

- **Patters** – Probably the simplest form of physical compassion approved by the American Medical Association. This is when the doctor stands next to the parent, usually at the patient's crib and makes soft repetitious pats on the parent's shoulder. Like patting the family dog on the head, this action is always accompanied with some sort of positive verbal comment. This word and action combo meal act like an epoxy bonding agent and helps with the quality of the closing statement.

• **Rubbers** – Borrowing from the Mr. Miagi art form of circular rotation, the doctors rub the parent's shoulders in a clockwise fashion. This professional contact shows feelings of concern as well as to help lull the parent into a trance. Keep in mind that with a comatose parent there is no need for any further verbal comments. Think "Wax on wax off."

• **Tappers** – When I happen to be sitting next to Zachary's crib during rounds the doctor will often pull up a chair to discuss the day's planned events. During this fireside chat they explain the day's plan of attack using their clipboard or bedside monitor as a visual aid. Upon their exit they will tap the parent's thigh twice to reinforcement the deep connection between the two parties. Never once mind you but twice! Three times would be just too weird.

• **Punchers** – Usually from a male doctor, this action is done from a standing position away from the crib. The doctor, whom I suspect has watched lots of Rocky movies, will opt to end his conversation with some sort of simulated single punch to the arm. Keep in mind that this is strictly a testosterone filled manly action that if happened to be done outside the hospital would have been followed by spitting on the ground.

So while Deanna and I hang with Zachary taking turns holding the little guy we wait for the doctors to round and discuss his health. In the meantime we will flip the channels on the overhead television.

> *Hey, looks like Karate Kid is on channel 4.*
>
> *Brian & Deanna*

Blog: Blood Type

Submitted 3/11/2008

At an early age I remember watching all of the science fiction shows from The Jetsons, Quantum Leap and Star Wars to name a few. All of these programs gave us a glimpse of what was in store for the human race. It was all very exciting with the personal robots, flying cars and space boots that everyone seemed to wear. Yes, the future seems so cool and advanced. Every day it seems, we inch a little closer to that future.

When Zachary was diagnosed with NEC (Necrotizing Enterocolitis) I was thrown into the future world of medicine. I learned so many things about the human body and how the medical community can step in and repair damage. Eye opening? Shocked? Amazed? All understatements. It appears as though the future had arrived in the hospitals a tad faster than any Jedi knight could muster. It seems that nothing was impossible.

Almost nothing.

Case in point: the other day I had one of those brief hallway chats with the transplant doctor. This is the kind of conversation that only happens when two people meet in the middle of an isolated corridor and some sort of verbal chit chat is expected. The doc tells me that things are looking up for Zachary as they see signs of activity in Children's transplant department. "How's that?" I inquired. He tells me that just last week there were two sets of organs from infants that would have fit Zachary just fine except they were of the blood type "B".

B! "Well, why couldn't that work?" I wondered as Zachary's blood type is A positive. Surely such a close match should be doable. Heck, I was told that Zachary could use organs with blood type "O" and that is waaaaaaaaay farther down the alphabet line than "B". Isn't there some sort of drug that allows for blood types that are close enough? It's not like the organs were blood type "T". We're talking "B". That's only one letter difference.

When you've been waiting for organs as long as us, this argument actually makes sense.

So even though the doctors can replace a defective liver, a worn intestinal tract and a less than perfect stomach – all before noon, they can't sidestep one letter in Zachary's blood type. I asked the doctor if there was any harm in trying. He just gave me a stare and walked away. Apparently he didn't take me seriously.

Probably a good thing that I'm not in the medical profession.

Brian & Deanna

Blog: The Next 24 Hours

Submitted 3/16/2008

Ever have one of those days when you wake up and just don't feel right? It is hard to explain but the source of your irritation could simply be a stomach ache. Then again it could be something south of the stomach. Perhaps a cramp in the calf muscle has migrated its way to the belly area. Kinda like the Single Bullet Theory. Whatever the case, you just know that something isn't right and all you can really do is lie on the couch, watch videos and moan. Perhaps consume a Big Gulp of your favorite beverage and a box of Pop Tarts.

This is a loose approximation of what is going on with Zachary this week. Medically speaking he appears to be in fine shape. His lab results are no different than before. He is getting all of the proper nutrients. He is getting more than enough sleep. Yet Zachary is just in some sort of bad mood.

A few days ago we noticed a few additional issues materializing. First, his heart rate started inching upwards. No reason why really. At least no reason that made sense. Then his blood pressure started to drop. Again, there were no blatant and obvious explanations. The doctors thought that maybe Zachary had too much fluid in his chest cavity and tried diuretics. This only worsened the blood pressure problem. Then they compensated by giving him some saline solutions in hope of raising his blood pressure to something more favorable. It helped the blood pressure but hindered his breathing issues.

What to do? What to do? What to do?

The rule of thumb in the hospital it seems is when a patient needs specialized one-on-one care then they really should be in the PICU – which luckily for us specializes in this type of one-on-one care. This way the patient has a designated nurse whose sole job is to take care of a single patient and answer all of my insanely odd and off-the-wall questions.

So as of Sunday morning Zachary was transferred to the PICU. Actually this was the first time that Deanna and I suggested (rather strongly too) the move. Like expected, Zachary is getting highly attentive care and the results are already showing. So far, his respiratory issues are starting to get under control. His heart rate is normal and blood pressure, although on the low end of normal, is starting to creep up.

Now that Zachary's PICU doctor is getting some of the issues out of the panic mode she is starting to figure out just what started this whole dilemma in the first place. You gotta love those A-type personalities. They are always thinking ahead. Let's hope that it is something as simple as the common cold. Unfortunately we have to consider the other unfavorable options like pneumonia or *a bacterial infection. No better place to catch a bug than in the hospital.*

The doctor says that the next 24 hours will tell them a lot. All I know is that this next day is going to be a long day.

Brian & Deanna

Blog: *The Past 24 Hours*
Submitted 3/17/2008

It's been a long day and an even longer night. There was very little sleep for Deanna and myself as we worried about Zachary and his apparent free fall from stability. Lots of activity, mostly bad, occurred last night after Deanna left the PICU. It was stressful to hear the phone ring in the middle of the night but at the same time you want to know what is going on. It is a double edged sword and we are getting cut from both sides.

Zachary is back on the ventilator on modest settings as his ability to breath was becoming more and more difficult. It seems that there was a fluid buildup in his lungs that the diuretics just wasn't able to reduce. Unfortunately this was the highlight of his night. Liver readings have skyrocketed. Figures like INR (a coagulation factor) which have already been high at 2.5 (normal is 1.0) have risen to an unprecedented 4.5. Honestly, I didn't know that it was possible to get that high.

The kidneys are taking a beating too. This could be due to the previous week's gameplan to dry Zachary out. Without ample fluid in his body the kidneys don't have anything to filter. At this point, it may be necessary to hydrate his body to help the kidneys and accept the fact that other problems will most certainly develop.

His platelet count, white blood cell and red blood cell count have all tanked. So to compensate the doctors have begun appropriate transfusions in hope of helping Zachary to battle some of these deficiencies. His blood pressure, which just 12 hours ago was showing signs of improvement have dropped. This has necessitated the use of blood pressure assisted drugs (Epinephrine, NorEpinephrine). This alone will probably drop us out of the picture for organs - for now that is.

Bacterial cultures were taken in hopes of getting some idea of the reason behind this huge drop. So far, nothing is showing positive. Keep in mind that these cultures can take up to five days to show a positive sign. If something shows positive within 24 hours, then the thought is that the virus or bacteria is running rampant in the blood stream. The longer the tests take to show a positive sign means a weaker population in the blood. So, the fact that nothing has shown up this early is somewhat comforting. But just in case something is brewing, various antibiotics have been given.

Although to early to know for sure the current theory points to pneumonia. In fact, Zachary was still showing signs of recovery from this same viral infection from his last encounter back on January 21. If things were ever worse for Zachary I can't remember when. He is a strong little kid and I'm hopeful that he will do whatever it takes to pull through. His resume is pretty good in this category.

Let's all keep Zachary in your thoughts.

Brian & Deanna

Blog: Turn the Band

Submitted 3/21/2008

Deanna and I were at the hospital gift shop the other day looking at some toys to put into Aidan's & Zachary's Easter basket. There were lots of plastic windup trucks and other toys with lights and sounds - always a winning combination for children under the age of five. In addition to these cheap Chinese imports I found a small kaleidoscope and instinctively gave it a visual try. With each turn of the band, it gave me a whole new vantage point of the different crystals and colors. Another turn and a completely different look.

This is a good way to describe Zachary's present condition. There are so many things going on, each with their own level of progress that determining his overall situation is a lot like looking through the kaleidoscope. As each hour passes the medical picture changes just like turning the band.

Let me shed some light on Zac's current condition. Due to the damage caused by the Strep Pneumonia virus a tremendous amount of fluids and blood products were needed to be given to our son. This caused his body to inflate a tremendous amount. In normal patients the kidneys would recognize this increase in water weight and respond by increased urine output. With liver failure patients, the kidneys tend not to function that well and the water stays in the body. The end result is that internal organs like the lungs cannot expand to their desired size which in turn causes his respiratory system to compromise their ability to work effectively.

With liver failure patients there is a long list of problems that tend to develop in addition to these situations. And in Zachary's case, it is a long list. If this isn't enough, we just found out this morning that another type infection was found in his Broviac line. The Broviac line is the main source of input for intravenous fluids, medicines and other types of drugs. Another infection changes everything.

Turn the band.

It seems that we have taken several steps back in Zachary's treatment. As some of his clotting factors have increased to a level of concern the doctors felt that some sort of dialysis was needed. This action would require the insertion of two catheters, one for blood in one for blood out and thus another trip down to the surgery room. The doctors wanted to prolong this intervention as long as possible due to other associated complications like bleeding, additional sources of infection, etc...

Of course there is Zachary's fluid overload situation to consider too. There was hope that his kidneys could be forced to excrete water with the aid of diuretics. This plan worked well for awhile but other factors like decreased blood pressure diminished this effectiveness.

Turn the band.

So in the end the catheter was the way to go. This new game plan would, in theory, allow for the waste removal of toxins in the blood as well as a way to take out fluid from Zachary. Now for some reason Zachary's blood pressure has stepped up a notch which has in turn increased his urine production. This out-of-the-blue turn of events has allowed the doctors to put off the dialysis. For now that is.

Turn the band.

So Deanna and my role today is to hang out by Zachary's crib and wait for something to change. It seems to be the only thing that we can count on. That and play with his Easter basket toys.

Brian & Deanna

Blog: Youth and Maturity

Submitted 3/25/2008

Back when I was in the fifth grade and sporting some cool bell bottom jeans I remember getting together with some other classes in the gymnasium and hearing about poor people in Africa. The teacher had some UNICEF volunteers who showed us pictures of other African kids about our age as well as photos of their small huts that they lived in. Thinking back I think that the teacher wanted us to feel some sort of appreciation for our own lives and perhaps help the needy sub Saharan people. To the best of my recollection I did neither.

It's not that I was a bad kid. I just had other things to think about. Dodge ball was big back then and thus I probably had that on my mind. I'm sure there may have been some math homework or an episode of Wonder Woman that evening that made me forget about anyone not in my class, on my bus or on my baseball team. Even in fifth grade I was thinking in terms of social circles.

I'd like to think that over the years I've grown in character as an individual, a husband and a father. I make it a point to throw change in the Salvation Army's holiday kettle (providing that the bell ringer makes a reasonable attempt to look like Santa). I gave for Katrina victims and I ALWAYS buy those Thin Mints from the Girls Scouts.

Since the COTA web site has been up and running Deanna and I have been surprised, shocked, overwhelmed...I'm not really sure of the best term to use here. Whatever the verbiage, we are constantly reminded just how Zachary has touched the lives of young people. These kids...or more appropriately young adults have helped to raise funds in support of my family.

Many of these fundraising stories for Zachary have certainly changed Deanna and my perception of youth and generosity for these very amazing young people. Some day I hope to meet up with these kids and thank them for a maturity that was way above any bar that I set at that age.

In my own defense though, Wonder Woman did get some high television ratings.

Brian & Deanna

Blog: Lottery Prediction

Submitted 3/27/2008

The Pennsylvania lottery was up to $270 million a few weeks ago. With this financial motivation I scrounged up a few dollars from my collection of quarters hiding under my car seat and bought a few tickets. I had dreams of winning it big and passed my time commuting from the apartment to the hospital thinking of how I would allocate this abundance of cash. Unfortunately this new life that I was hoping for was not to be as I did not have the five winning numbers. For that matter I did not have even one number. Granted the chances of me picking all five numbers are pretty high. But how depressing is it to miss all five numbers?

In spite of the odds (1 in 14 million for you statisticians) they seem much better than my attempts at predicting Zachary's health. In spite of all of the information that I have learned about pediatrics over the past 20 months I routinely get it wrong when trying to anticipate Zachary's medical trends.

Let's step back in time a little shall we? The last few weeks were not kind for Zachary. He was transferred back to the PICU, fought off two infections, was placed on the ventilator to assist him in his breathing issues and gained over three liters of fluids in the form of blood products, medicines, antibiotics solutions, TPN (daily liquid nutrients) and a few pints of 10-W40 for good measure. The end result was a very puffy Zachary, somewhat high ventilator settings, less than promising chest x-rays, and some concern of ongoing heart failure.

Understandably my prediction of his health was a little on the doom-and-gloom side. With all of these issues on the table I was less than optimistic of his short term goals. I did not think that Zachary would pull it together short of three weeks. Again I was proven wrong.

First of all the doctors concentrated on his fluid problems. They placed him on diuretics to kick start his kidneys into doing their job. Slowly at first, the kidneys started to filter out the abundance of water in Zachary's tissues. When the doctors felt comfortable with this they increased the diuretics and the kidneys picked up the pace. As of today Zachary's water retention level is very minimal.

His infection has been beaten back and appears to be gone. His breathing issues have been tempered and if all goes well today (knock on wood), Zachary will be off of the ventilator and breathing on his own. As far as additional blood products, a nominal amount to be transfused is normal for liver failure kids. It seems that Zachary is slowly getting back to this nominal amount.

The bottom line is that Zachary is back on the transplant list. His issues have been corrected over the past 10 days - far better and faster than I anticipated. As his condition improves Deanna and I tend to sleep better too. With this said, the past few days have seen some hibernation type sleep patterns for Mom and Dad.

With some sleep under my belt I tend to think more clearly. Perhaps now I can better predict Zachary's health over the next few weeks. With this increased brain power I may be better able to predict the winning lottery numbers.

I just wonder if there are any more quarters under my car seat.

Brian & Deanna

Blog: Dream of a Life
Submitted 4/02/2008

It's 4:30pm on a Wednesday here in Children's PICU. I recently commandeered a comfortable rocking chair and placed it within an arm's reach of Zachary's crib. My responsibility today is to watch my son breath in and out and wait for the best time to pick him up for some Daddy snuggle time. Personally I would rather hold him all the time but I know that his sleep is very important too. Of course, he has been sleeping a lot over the past two weeks.

Should I wake him now?

Should I let him rest?

As I contemplate this decision my mind wanders and I look around the PICU. It seems that all of the nurses this shift has spent some time with Zachary. Deanna and I know most all of their names, if they are married or single, where they live, if they have kids or pets. Just like in any office environment, some of these workers are better than others. Even though the talent bar is set high in the PICU we have our favorites.

Looking around I have to admit that the PICU is an odd place to hang out. There is the constant foot traffic of personnel, the bright lights and the alarms of pumps going off at most every second. Kinda reminds me of the casinos in Vegas. The accommodations in the PICU are cramped as there is not much extra room in this space controlled ward. Thankfully we are located in a corner unit which allows our various machines to spread over into other areas.

Looking over at Zachary I am reminded that he has an upward march to complete in order to get back out of the PICU. His latest battle with pneumonia left him weak. He is not moving his arms as much and will open his eyes on limited occasions. We take this brief opportunity to communicate, read books and move his arms and legs up and down. Every little bit helps.

On a positive note, Zachary was extubated yesterday. This means that the tube that was originally inserted through his mouth and down into his lungs was removed. The tube was originally placed to provide Zac with ample breathing assistance. As he showed some increased strength in this area the decision was made to remove the tube and let him breath on his own. It was not a clear cut decision though as his breathing is not really that strong and thus the doctors may have to reinsert the tube (aka intubate) at any given time. Consider it a medical roll of the dice.

Recently I spoke to the transplant doctors regarding what kind of organs they would consider for Zachary when the time comes. Originally they were holding out for organs from a smaller child. Organs of a smaller size, they state, would fit within Zachary chest cavity and allow for anticipated swelling as they sutured the post transplant opening.

As time has gone by these parameters have been widened to include children 2 to 3 times Zachary's size. This less preferred route would make it difficult to suture up the abdomen with the larger organs and swelling. To compensate some sort of synthesized temporary skin would be needed until Zachary grew into the space. So even though this is not the idea route it is now on the table as an option.

I look back at Zachary. He looks comfortable and breathing easier. Maybe I'll let him sleep a while longer. Let him dream of a life outside of the hospital.

He certainly has earned it.

Brian & Deanna

Blog: Around the Bend

Submitted 4/05/2008

Every day, it seems, one of the hospital's social workers will stop by to see how things are going. From what I can tell their job to provide parents with some level of support ranging from parking passes, meal tickets or simply a shoulder to lean on. Barring a stiff drink, there seems to be a wide swatch of support at their fingertips.

Not too long ago the social worker stopped by as I was at Zachary's cribside and quickly realized that what I really needed was just to be left alone. Upon leaving she suggested a good movie with lots of popcorn. She got half of it right.

So a few weeks later I took this advice, played couch potato and flipped through my cable box programs to watch the movie Braveheart. It was a great flick if you like violence, rebellious acts against authority, and the chance to root against the underdog. The best part of the film though, is the "Give One For The Gipper" speech that Mel Gibson's character orates to the hundreds of Scottsmen gathered for the battle - all while riding back and forth on a horse. Ah, the talents that some people possess. It was a well written speech that rounded up the troops and gave them inspiration to go out and kick lots of British butt.

As a sidenote I always wondered how everyone on the front battle line heard the entire speech considering that Mel's character didn't have any type of loudspeaker or sound system nearby. Surely the rank and file would have missed some of the pertinent points of his awe inspiring rhetoric. "Excuse me Mr. Braveheart, can you repeat that last part? Me and Shamus didn't hear a word down here."

Okay, so where am I going with this? Just stay patient and continue reading. I'll tie this in somehow.

As parents of a transplant-to-be patient there is no room for down time. You really have to be there 100% for your child no matter what the daily blood tests show. Whether it is the mornings, weekends or holidays the Parenthood Manual clearly requires mandatory attendance each and every day. The manual also covers such subjects as upbeat and optimistic thoughts, ample supply of Baby Einstein videos and of course, colorful balloons. There are no exceptions to these rules. No passes. No variances.

In spite of the clear cut etched-in-stone set of rules, it seems that, from time to time Deanna and I may drop our energy level a notch or two. It's not that we lose faith in Zachary's ability to rebound from infections or even our confidence in the medical staff. Not at all. Like any parent we just need to take a deep breath, regroup, and move forward with today's events.

Sometimes you have to be able to look beyond today's situation and visualize how things will be tomorrow. You have to be able to look down the road and see around the bend. Consider it a sixth sense. Looking around curves is one of those hidden powers that parallels parenthood. Superman, Batman, the X-Men have nothing on us. They just have better costumes. Still, no one told Deanna and I how difficult this was going to be.

Perhaps it is our turn to line up on Scottish side of the battle line. Maybe we should take a turn at the back end of a motivational speech from someone with a blue painted face and accent. Maybe the social worker can arrange for this type of thing in the PICU on Monday. Just like in the movie.

Minus the horse.

Brian & Deanna

Blog: Hence the Bleeding

Submitted 4/08/2008

The other day started off in the normal way. Upon walking up to Zachary's crib Deanna saw a rather cute and stable child lying peacefully all snuggled up in a blue and white blanket. This is the kind of visual that makes you want to break out the camera and take a few photos for Grandma and Grandpa. The moment, though, was short lived.

For no apparent reason Zachary started to bleed from his mouth. Wave after wave of blood was spit up and pooled alongside his neck. All of the nearby gauze was used to contain the mess but the blood just kept coming. It was a scary site but Deanna, along with the nurse, cleaned the blood and suctioned out the remaining red fluids in Zachary's mouth.

For such a scary situation, there was an amazing order of calmness. How long the bleeding would continue was unknown. What to do to keep this from happening again was unknown as well. The visual imagery was compelling for sure but it needed to be set aside for now. A line was crossed. Zachary was getting sicker. It was time for answers.

Two days later we have only limited information on the source of the bleed. It could have originated in the intestinal tract. Then again it could be the throat area. Using some sort of scope or camera to view this area may solve the problem but then again this procedure could cause additional bleeding. So the scope approach was vetoed. The best course of action is to beef up the coagulation factors by transfusing Zachary with lots and lots of platelets and other blood products.

It is the thought of the doctors that Zac's liver has taken another hit. His ability to clot blood is compromised even more. To counter this situation the doctors are inundating Zachary with all kinds of blood products to give him the ability to form clots. From what we were told it is a natural progression of liver failure to lose this clotting ability.

What prompted the liver's drop has been blamed on yet another infection - the second time in a week. Technically, the doctors tell us that the infection has prompted the walls in his intestinal tract to become perforated or leaky... hence the bleeding. So although the increased transfusions will slow the bleeding somewhat, the infection will have to be taken care of to stop the bleeding entirely.

At the end of this day Zachary is still sedated in his crib lying calmly and comfortably. The bleeding has been slowed waaaay down. He is on the ventilator and a few more antibiotics running around his arteries and veins. His blood pressure, heart rate, temperature are all stable. At times he opens his eyes and reaches for his teddy bear.

From the outside things look stable. Unfortunately for Zachary, the inside is what counts. So in the meantime we continue to wait for a donor.

The waiting can be excruciating.

Brian & Deanna

Blog: Perspective

Submitted 4/18/2008

I guess that it is simply a matter of perspective on how Zachary looks. A fresh face would no doubt fumble for words to describe him. As parents, we have learned to overlook the façade and concentrate on the inside. How is the blood pressure? What is his ammonia level? Are Zachary's kidney's working well? What does it take to keep him in the running for organ transplant? These are the areas that we are focusing on.

It is not like we are oblivious to the obvious physical signs. It is kinda hard to over look this from anyone's vantage point – even more from a parent. Still, we know that his puffiness is not at the top of the list of concerns. We realize that the bruises on his skin (caused by poor coagulation factors) will go away another day. His orange skin will be gone when the transplant is completed. It's an acquired ability to look past these traits of your child and concentrate on more important issues.

It's not always easy to segment these issues.

But we have developed a routine to our visits. In the morning upon arriving we enter the PICU, wash our hands and head for Zachary's crib. Standing beside our son we do a quick visual inspection complete with some hand holding, kisses or a brief pep talk. At this point we turn our attention to the above monitor. How is his heart rate? What is his blood pressure? Is he getting enough oxygen in his blood?

The next step in our routine is to look at the various pumps surrounding the crib. Has his sedation drug gone up? Gone done? How much blood pressure medicine is he getting? What is the status with blood products? The final leg of this research trilogy are the labs. After grabbing Zac's chart we look at his ammonia levels, blood coagulation figures and sodium numbers to list a few. With this type of information we discuss his status with the nurse and doctors.

It is not the easiest thing to disconnect your feelings as a parent and review the numbers. But at the same time it is crucial to know what is going on. Sometimes you keep the emotions in check and other times you don't.

Currently we see that Zachary's condition is improved from the other day. He still has some bleeding in his intestinal tract which is causing some issues with high ammonia and low blood levels. The doctor's plan to increase his platelet count to combat this problem seems to be working. Zachary's ability to fight off the infection looks to be going well too. His water overload situation is gradually getting better as the arrangement of different diuretics is slowly gaining ground. This in turn helps his breathing issues.

Yes, the situation is better but we know from prior experience (both in the past and recent) that things can change within the hour. However, I must once again state that I'm amazed just how much fighting stamina this little guy has.

No matter what the perspective.

Brian & Deanna

Blog: Shades of Gray

Submitted 4/15/2008

Lately it has become somewhat difficult to accurately convey the status of Zachary's health. There are just so many nuances to his overall medical picture that frankly I don't know where to start. I guess it is on par to describing shades of gray. The hardest part is knowing where to start. So in this blog I am going to ramble from the middle and spread outwards.

Three weeks ago Zachary caught strep pneumonia. A week later he tested positive for the Klebsiella infection. These bugs are not kind to kids of any age. They can make the healthiest of toddlers sick enough for a trip to the hospital. In Zachary's case the effect has been nearly disastrous.

At the moment Zachary's blood pressure is very weak and requires the assistance of the drug NorEpidepherine. Each day he seems to be on the losing end of the battle as more and more of this drug is needed to keep his blood pressure stable. His breathing too is very weak and is supported by a ventilator machine.

Because of the high settings of this machine there was a tendency for Zachary to resist the machine's breathing rhythms. Since fighting this machine wasn't helping the healing process it became necessary to sedate and paralyze him. The process has helped Zachary to breath easier but it is not by any means foolproof. His right lung collapses on occasion which requires still higher settings.

As the liver continues to lose functionality many electrolytes are getting out of whack. Currently the doctors are battling daily low levels like calcium and potassium as well as high levels of ammonia and sodium. Each one of these can cause some serious problems ranging from seizures to heart problems.

If this wasn't enough Zachary is still battling a water weight issue. When things got bad he needed additional fluids to keep his blood pressure stable. Of course, stable blood pressure comes with a price. In Zachary's case these extra fluids settled in his lungs which in turn caused more breathing issues. It's a Catch 22.

It gets worse.

It has come to the attention of the neurology doctors that a prior bleeding spell has somehow pooled blood into the area between the brain and skull. The neurologist tells us that this type of problem should involve surgery before any talk of transplant. Currently we are getting a second (and third) opinion on this but either way if it isn't the first priority then I'm sure that it is certainly a close second.

So Zachary's greatest challenge now is not improving his breathing ability. It is not strengthening his blood pressure or even brain surgery. His greatest challenge is buying more time for his liver.

It is crunch time. The 11th hour. The two minute warning.

What more can I say?

Brian & Deanna

Blog: One More Day

Never Submitted

At night I walk the hospital hallways. One arm holds a small boy clinging onto a life that he barely knows. The other arm pulls along his lifeline of medical pumps, antibiotics and life sustaining fluids that keeps him going for another day. At times the hallway is empty and I feel an uneasy aloneness with my son. I hope for smiles. I settle for anything really. All I ask for is one more day.

Deanna and I have traded in our comfortable lives in Severna Park, Maryland for a small apartment near the hospital. Zachary's twin brother Aidan, Deanna and myself are putting our lives on hold while we balance hope and the realities of transplant life every day. The health of Zachary is the major force that keeps us going. His good days are our good days. When his health slips a little piece of us goes along with him. It's not a partnership we expected when he was born. But then again life is not fair.

Like many of the parents of this wing we are waiting for donor organs. In Zachary's case he needs a liver and small intestine. The availability of such organs is rare. Because of his small size the availability of such a commodity is even rarer. Even though his advanced liver failure has put him at the top of the national list we are constantly reminded that this doesn't guarantee results. We have been waiting six months and the wait continues. Time is not on our side.

Our jobs have been left behind. Our house is vacant. Our dog is staying with relatives in Ohio.

Money is tight. Stress is high. Our health is at best compromised.

Through out it all, our main focus is keeping a family together in a place that we don't want to be. We want to be home. We want our family intact. We want our lives back.

However tonight we will settle for walking the hospital hallways one more time.

Brian & Deanna

Chapter 16

How   Transplantation   Works

A few weeks after Zachary's arrival to Children's he was deemed healthy enough to be placed on the Liver / Bowel transplant list. This is a national list that assigns some sort of order to those recipients waiting for the availability of organs. This list gives priorities to the sickest patients (but not to sick) within a region and then to the sickest patients (but not to sick) on a national level. Many patients often do spend large amounts of time waiting it out for available organs. Unfortunately, many patients die while waiting it out. It is a sad reality of life that there is more demand than supply. This was a possibility that the transplant doctors made certain that we were aware of.

Once you are on the list you feel a little better about the situation. Meaning you feel that your child finally has a chance at a renewed lease on life. You know whether it is during the day or in the middle of the night you may get a call from the transplant team. It is a call that you hope happens sooner rather than later. In our case sooner came and went. Later was knocking on the door.

There are many reasons why Zachary was waiting for so long for available organs. One of the biggest reasons was his health. Even though he was healthy enough to get a transplant doesn't mean that just any set of organs will do. In other words, if Zachary was really healthy then the transplant doctors could be a little more liberal on the quality of the donor organs. But seeing as he is a very sick patient, not to mention a very sick transplant candidate patient, there is no margin for anything less than perfect-conditioned organs. Hence, Zachary needed the best organs that he could get.

During this time of waiting we heard rumors that organs became available often. We would get all excited and then learn that the organs were either the wrong size or the organs were from a patient who wasn't very healthy before their death. It never seemed to be an ideal match. As time passed and Zachary's condition deteriorated Deanna and I had several meetings with the transplant doctors. We tried to persuade them to loosen their requirements a little but each time they held their ground and insisted on waiting for the best organs. Their reasons were, as always, sound and logical but as time passed Deanna and I cared less about their reasons. We had our own reasons. We wanted Zachary to live.

Now, obtaining organs isn't as simple as visiting your local Organ Depot store. First of all, we tried the living donor approach. This is where organs are taken from an ideal match like a parent or sibling of adult age. Before we even got out of the gate in asking the question this idea was dismissed. The Children's doctors felt that operating on either Deanna or myself posed too much risk in obtaining organs for Zachary.   So this left us with only one other option. In order for Zachary to live, someone else had to die.

Plain and simple.

No one wants to obtain organs this way but frankly speaking, there is no other way. It's a tough condition to accept but one we had to come to grips with.

As each day passed and we waited desperately for donor organs we started to put more weight on various dates on the calendar. We learned from the ICU nurses that certain times of the year tend to yield more fatalities than others. For instance, the Memorial Day weekend means that pools open for the public. Open pools; unfortunately mean more drownings and thus possible donor organs.

When a nice weekend is forecasted it usually translates into more children visiting the ICU with bicycle accidents. This too could mean possible donor organs. Halloween is another time of the year where there is a spike in accidents. As kids, gowned in dark costumes, dart out in front of cars the result often is a trip to the hospital. Again, there is the chance of possible donor organs.

We learned that one of the leading causes of deaths among teenagers in the state of Pennsylvania are All Terrain Vehicles (ATVs) and motocross accidents. I became friends with a father of a teenager who was in the PICU for just this reason. The son was a talented motocross rider who tried to jump his bike a little too high on a turn and ended up injuring his neck. Standing near Zachary's crib and overlooking his son the father said that his teenager's competitive motocross days were now over. He also confided that he should have made this decision one day earlier.

Last I heard, the young teenager managed to survive the ordeal. Although he was one of the lucky survivors of a motocross neck injury he will be dealing with the aftermaths of the accident for many years to come.

Deanna and I learned that stricter seatbelt laws and better child restraints have resulted in lower auto fatalities for young children. No one can argue that this is a bad thing but try telling that to a parent whose own child is running out of time waiting for organs. So as the days passed we looked at Halloween, Memorial Day and the weather forecasts with a much different perspective.

Even though someone else's tragedy may occur doesn't necessarily mean that it will benefit Zachary. There are conditions that need to be met in order for Zachary to receive organs. Consider the following:

- Blood type needs to be a match. The preferred type of the donor would be Zachary's blood type of A Positive but if the situation became dire a universal donor blood type of O would be considered.
- Size of the donor's organs is very important, as there is only so much room within Zachary's abdomen. Since Zachary was weighing in at around 10 kilograms (22.2 lbs) the Transplant

team was hoping for a donor weight of 12 kilograms (26.4 lbs) or under.
• Cause of death of the donor must be taken into consideration. Cancer for instance would most certainly nullify the organs transfer as would issues like infections and/or blood pressure related problems. As callous as this sounds, an ideal cause of death would be some sort of head trauma resulting in the absence of brain activity coupled with little or no interruption of the circulatory system.
• Of course nothing would happen if the parents of the donor refused consent to donate the organs. Throughout such a traumatic experience this is not an easy topic for discussion as the family's thoughts are obviously on their child. No matter how bad the timing may appear, the question of organ donation needs to be approached if another child can be saved.

Donating our own organs upon death seems to be more common nowadays. It is as easy as checking the option box on your driver's license. Many of us don't think twice about this. After all, we feel that upon our death we won't be needing the organs so what's the harm. However, discussing this subject with your children's organs in mind somehow takes on a whole new perspective. Yet this is exactly the conversation that Deanna and I have made. It would by hypocritical of us to not consider it. Based on what we have experienced it would be wrong if we didn't agree to it. I is our hope that other parents agree to it as well.

Twice during this excruciating wait for organs we received phone calls from the Transplant team. On both occasions they had found what appeared to be ideal organs. Deanna and I were shocked and excited all at the same time. The doctors told us upfront that they still had to physically view the organs to determine if the quality was up to their standards.

The first time this happened we waited all through the night for confirmation of the healthy organs. This call, for one reason or another never came. I suspect that through the late night flight someone forgot to call the parents.

The second time things were different. We waited throughout the night and into the next morning. In spite of several phone calls from us no one at the PICU had heard anything suggesting that the organs were low quality. When we arrived at the hospital we were informed that Zachary had been taken to the OR for prepping. It seems that the transplant was a "Go" after all.

Then as fast as it began it ended. Within minutes of hearing the good news the phone rang and we found out that the donor organs were not high quality. This second time around was like the first. We were deflated, crushed and exhausted. In spite of the emotional let down, giving up was not an option.

Back to the PICU we went once again.

Chapter 17

Fundraising

The decision to temporarily relocate to Pittsburgh didn't take much thought. After all, Zachary's life depended on this transplant. Pittsburgh was a no brainer and a slam-dunk decision. But moving to the Steel City did pose a whole lot of problems – including financial. But not to worry though as we had a plan. Now that I think about it, we had a plan for about every occasion ranging from balancing credit card payments with debit cards to what to do when we ran out of skim milk during dinner. If there was one thing that we were good at, it was planning.

Obviously we were going to lose the full time job aspect and the income that went with it. It looked as if part time income was going to be in Vogue for us for the time being. In order to keep up with paying the bills on this new budget Deanna and I figured that if we could live on Spam and a side order of macaroni & cheese then perhaps this would be possible.

But after a short amount of time the reality of working part time in Maryland proved to be too much to handle. First of all the five hour commute time was difficult to deal with not to mention the cost of gas. For every day that Deanna and I were in Maryland necessitated having one of the Grandparents there to pick up the slack with Aidan. It soon became too much to ask.

It was time for Plan B.

So Deanna (always thinking ahead) searched out some fundraising web sites and came across a non-profit site called COTA (Center for Organ Transplant Association). This non-profit organization had helped hundreds of families in organizing fund raising projects and thus helped many families keep their homes in the process.

The process involved a grass roots effort of friends to basically raise money for the cause. It was a lot to ask of people who had families of their own as well as the normal time-consuming day-to-day activities but we felt that this was our best and only option. In other words, there was no Plan C.

We had asked four friends to take on this endeavor. All of these friends lived in the Severna Park area of which only one had prior fund raising experience. In the end it didn't seem to matter as they did a fantastic job of raising funds and in the process shared Zachary's story with hundreds if not thousands of people. The plan basically was for this team of four to pretty much do it all. Deanna and my role were limited to those of second-string cheerleaders. The idea behind cutting Deanna and me out of the loop was to allow us to focus all of our attention on Zachary.

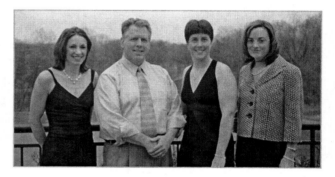

Fundraising volunteers from left: Kate, Josh, Debbie & Christine

Our team of four filled in the following slots:

- Kate, Trustee

With COTA staff, coordinated payment of patient bills and invoices.
- Josh, Public Relations Coordinator

Coordinated all media contacts, press releases and publicity for fundraising activities and events.
- Debbie, Campaign Coordinator

Oversaw all campaign activities and supervised committee chairpersons.
- Christine, Webmaster

Maintained and updated patient campaign website.

It didn't take long for this team to roll up their sleeves and get down to work. They started off small. A bake sale was set up at the local grocery store where they had hoped to net around $500. Of course it helped that some Public Relations work was done ahead of time. Lots of publicity was generated regarding "Home Town Zac" through both word of mouth as well as local press coverage. Once the momentum began it was hard to stop. When the bake sale was all said and done and the money was tallied up the team netted over $5,000. Who ever heard of a bake sale netting five grand?

What was in those cakes and cookies?

The activities didn't stop there as our volunteers were just getting started. They planned several fundraising events each one successful and impressive. One of these events to note was a well-planned and orchestrated silent auction complete with wine sponsors, professional caterers and a live band all held at a local country club. They enlisted more volunteers from the area, more donations and more publicity. The end result was a tally of over $41,000.

One thing was obvious. We picked the right people for the job. Our group of volunteers, dubbed "Team Zac" just kept rolling. But as it turns out, they weren't the only players raising money for Zachary. Friends of ours in other states had their own ideas. A friend of the family created and sold bracelets. An acquaintance brought Zac's cause to his workplace and got the boss to match contributions.

Age wasn't a factor either. On a few occasions, a younger generation took center stage and jumped onto the fundraising bandwagon.

✓   Carson Brinegar of Millersville, MD celebrated his 8th birthday with 18 of his friends. Instead of receiving gifts, he asked his friends to donate money (over $400) to Zac's fund.

✓   Mary Mitchell, an 8-year-old local girl celebrated her birthday by asking her friends to bring presents for Zac and Aidan, rather than for herself. In addition to that, this entrepreneur also held another fundraiser in which she provided a dog-walking service in exchange for donations to Zac's fund. Both events totaled $500.

✓   The nursery, pre-K and Kindergarten classes at St. Martin's-in-the-Field School in Severna Park started a coin fundraiser and brought in over $1,000.

✓   Daisy Troop 1788 of Severna Park raised nearly $200.

And this is just what I know of. Of course there are hundreds of anonymous contributors who, after tuning in to Zachary's web site donated funds. From last count this section of funds totaled over $30,000.

Of course, this did not mean that Deanna and I could simply access these funds whenever we wanted or for whatever we wanted. There were strict guidelines on the use of these financial contributions. For starters, we had to incur the cost first and then with proper documentation (i.e. receipts) we would get reimbursed for the expense(s). As it stood, even the types of expenses were subject to levels of scrutiny. For instance, our housing costs were reimbursed as was our food, transportation expenses and utilities. Items like socks, batteries and hair cuts were not reimbursable.

Even though we were seeing a healthy financial balance sheet from generous contributors this didn't equate to lavish expenses. All reimbursable items had to have some tie to Zachary. Sadly enough, I was never able to fully establish a relationship between a 42 inch flat screen high-definition television and Zachary's mental development. Perhaps I should have gone with the "Star Trek is an educational show" angle. I'll know better next time.

Throughout it all, Deanna and I were overwhelmed by the generosity of so many people to the point where we just couldn't process it all. Many times I wondered what motivated complete strangers to open up their wallets and contribute money to Zachary's fund. Did there exist some sort of common thread that connected Zachary's story to the life of a stranger? I am sure that some of these people who contributed knew us but the vast majority, I suspect, had never even met us – or were probably not likely to either. How many people did his story touch?

This experience was certainly an eye-opening ordeal on many levels.

The commitment of friendship.

The maturity of children.

The generosity of strangers.

Chapter 18

I n s u r a n c e

I
n the old days it was love that made the world go round and round. In today's tough economic world it's a good insurance plan. Like a lot of men, we take a tremendous amount of time researching insurance for our cars but kinda skip through the handbook when it comes to health insurance. I guess we have this Superman mentality and figure that we are invincible. Blame it on testosterone.

After moving to Maryland, it was Deanna's part time employer who supplied our health benefits. From what I gathered, the benefits seemed fine. Of course, my barometer of a good plan involved a simple question. If I got hit by a bus would the insurance cover the damages and thus let me stay in my house? It was a basic question requiring a simple yes or no response. If the answer was yes then I didn't bother to read the policy handbook. If the question was no, I would have most certainly read the handbook ...but later...when I had nothing else going on. Keep in mind that the art of procrastination is a close relative of the Y chromosome.

Prior to the birth of the twins, insurance was the last thing on my mind. I was too busy thinking of other things like painting the walls in my house, trimming tree branches in the yard or where to get my hair cut. The mere fact that we had insurance was good enough for me. To the best of my knowledge I never even looked at the policy. The way I figured it, I had already done the research (reference the bus scenario).

However, things changed when Aidan and Zachary were born. Suddenly reading the insurance policy was more important than looking through my stack of unread This Old House magazines. I was now in sponge mode and wanted to know what health issue was covered and what wasn't. Suffice it to say this wasn't an easy task. The insurance policy writers don't make reading these documents something the average Joe could do. There were lots of words I didn't recognize which required me to read and reread everything. The learning curve had begun and it was a very slow process.

With Deanna filling in the role as an insurance translator I started to realize that she had a pretty good plan. In spite of all of the data on benefits thrown at me I must admit that I never really understood it all. But I understood enough. Zachary had a $2 million dollar cap. This means that our insurance plan paid for his surgeries, his overnight stays and even the countless diapers and sterile gauze bandages that he required. In other words, when it was all said and done and Zachary was sent home after his gut healed my family would still have a home to go to.

It seemed that $2 million of insurance was more than enough.

As the months passed and Zachary's condition failed to improve we continued to bounce our son in and out of the hospital. Somewhere around his first birthday the bills totaled over $600,000. We had learned enough about bowels and livers at this point to realize that there were two possible routes for recovery: Rehab or Transplant. Rehab was an expensive route but was becoming unlikely. Unfortunately the transplant route was even more expensive and was now gaining ground.

We learned that a liver / bowel transplant was the pricier of transplants costing around $500,000. At this point we started doing the math. A transplant would put us roughly over a million dollars and suddenly the $2 million cap appeared closing in on us very quickly. There weren't many options at this point to choose from and was all becoming very nightmarish. Would we have to sell our house? Then what?

Thankfully there was alternative plan. The state of Maryland adopted a program sometime ago called REM (Rare and Expensive

Medical Plan). This was an insurance program offered to both adults and adolescents with severe issues like mental disorders, spinal cord injuries, transplants, etc... This state program made it possible for Zachary's medical care to be covered after the $2 million cap was reached. It's a good thing that we were accepted as several months into Zachary's admittance to Children's Hospital of Pittsburgh we had reached that $2 million limit.

Keep in mind that we were totally grateful for the assistance for without this aid Deanna and I would have been forced to sell our house and live in a FEMA trailer in a flood zone for many years. However, being that this program is run by a state agency means that there were bound to be some...shall we say "miscommunications" along the way?

The REM program was intended to help Maryland residents with huge devastating events like, in Zachary's case, a transplant. But the program was intended to pay for these issues to a facility within the state's borders. Since Zachary's situation started in Maryland all was fine. As soon as he was airlifted to a facility in another state the policy became blurred. Initially we seemed to get a waiver of sorts for medical payments to out-of-state Children's.

However, as our son started to improve his condition and whispers of discharge began to emanate around the PICU we soon learned about the cracks in the system. It seemed that discharging Zachary to our temporary apartment in nearby Shadyside (Pittsburgh) was going against Maryland policy and thus Maryland Medicaid wasn't willing to fork over any money. They insisted that we move back to Maryland in order for payments to resume.

This is where the nightmare began. It seemed obvious that staying local was in Zachary's best interests. After all, if a call for a transplant materialized then we could simply put Zac in the car seat and drive him from our Shadyside apartment to Children's. Total commute time: 15 minutes. The state of Maryland though, would have required us to drive Zachary from our house in Maryland to

Children's. Total commute time: 5 hours. When organs have a limited shelf life outside of the host body this posed a major hurdle in the timing department.

So this left us with a few options – none of which looked promising.

1.   Stay in Pittsburgh and pay the bill ourselves; keeping in mind that neither Deanna nor myself had jobs and needed to be there for Zachary at any given moment.

2.   Move back to Maryland and plan on driving like maniacs when organs became available.

3.   Write a letter to influential Congress type people and plead our case. Perhaps request another waiver.

It didn't take much brainpower to figure out that Option #3 was the leading candidate. I wrote letters to various elected officials within Maryland's government and to my surprise actually received responses very quickly. The key to a fast response, it seems, was to mention that the problem revolves around a very sick child and more importantly that my blogs on the subject are being read by thousands of registered voters. In the end, for whatever the official reason, the policy was tweaked in Zachary's favor.

As it turned out, Zachary experienced an infection soon after this ordeal and was moved back to the PICU. The whispers of discharge never materialized and we continued our stay at Children's. All of this paperwork seemed to be in vain.

All sarcasm aside, the quickness of Maryland's elected officials to help us out in this financial crisis was quite impressive.   More importantly, we still had our house.

Chapter 19

The Call

Towards the middle of April 2008 Zachary's condition was not looking good. His blood results were continuously painting a bleak picture of his health. He was taking longer to rebound from infections and we were seeing routine signs of low blood pressure and various issues associated with his heart. Everyone knew that his health was wailing but at the same time nobody really wanted to say anything. It didn't matter really as their body language told us what we already knew. For the first time since Zachary's birth, Deanna and I had to accept the fact that our son may not make it. Knowing this fact paled in comparison to actually saying it out loud.

To make matters worse, Zachary had begun having brain seizures. No one knew what had caused this and sadly enough, no one really knew how to solve it. The timing of this couldn't have been worse. In order to eliminate the seizures, for the time being, was to medicate it away. Increasing Zachary's sedation didn't appear the best route but considering all of the other problems our son was experiencing this approach was the lesser of two evils.

With Zachary fully sedated, Deanna five months pregnant and both of us going without much needed rest we decided to give ourselves a break. Deanna would take Aidan up to her parent's in nearby Chardon (Cleveland), Ohio and regenerate her batteries for a few days. In the process, Aidan could run around the yard, play with our dog Bailey and in general wear out Grandma and Grandpa. I, on the other hand, would be able to visit Zachary, eat lots of pizza and watch as many episodes of South Park as I could find on our 120-channel cable box. It was essentially a three-day vacation from our lives.

Again, life intervened with alternate plans.

It was the middle of the night when I heard my cell phone ring. It could only mean one of two things. Either something very bad was happening with Zachary or something very good was about to happen to Zachary. In spite of the 50-50 split answering the phone still made me nervous. Whatever the case I was about to find out. It was time to pick up the phone.

"Hello" I said.

"We've got organs" the doctor stated.

I responded with overwhelming silence. It looks like Zachary was about to have something very good happen to him. I was excited and nervous all at the same time. This was the call that Deanna and I had been waiting for over the past year and it was happening now...at 3 in the morning...at the beginning of our three day "distressing vacation". I remembered that a friend of ours told us to expect this call when we least expected it – probably in the middle of the night. I guess she was right.

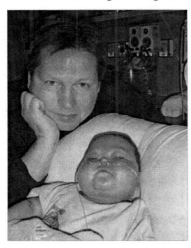

Brian with Zachary

I heard the rest of the conversation as clear as any phone call that I have ever had. The transplant doctor explained that he needed to fly out of state ASAP to view and procure the organs. He stated in bold print **that nothing was set in stone until that time**. But if all worked well then Zachary would be prepped and wheeled down to the Operating Room that morning, probably around 8am.

I called Deanna to spread the news. "Are you serious." she responded in the form of a statement.

To be honest, I was expecting a rather different response. Perhaps I didn't approach this topic of breaking news with a pregnant woman's sleep schedule in mind. But after a few seconds of realization we both shared the moment. Even though we knew that nothing was official, we had a feeling that this time it was going to happen.

That day everything seemed to happen according to someone else's clock. At 7am we got confirmation that the organs were good. Zachary was prepped by his nurse and was wheeled down to the Operating Room promptly at 8am. Upon leaving the PICU a crowd had gathered by the exit door consisting of those who had cared for Zachary over the months. Various doctors, nurses and therapists wanted to show their support on this very important event. Zachary's fan club, it seems, was seeing him off.

Deanna arrived at Children's at around 10am – much quicker than the speed limit allowed. The surgery lasted some 13 hours and was performed by two transplant doctors and a handful of support technicians and nurses. Over this time period Deanna and I chose to pass the time away from the hospital – hopefully keeping our minds off of the operation. We received cell phone updates every two hours from the Operating Room liaison and the surgeon himself. It was a big operation for sure but we were confident in the abilities of the surgeons. After all, they were the big reason why we came to Children's in the first place.

Later that night, after the surgery was finished the doctors gave Deanna and me a recount of Zachary's health as well as the highlights of his lengthy surgery. We were told that they replaced his liver, bowel, pancreas and stomach. Other organs taken out and not replaced included the spleen, gall bladder and appendix. When we inquired on this the docs told us that these last three organs were not essential to Zachary's recovery. It was unknown if we got some sort of credit on our bill for this organs - I decided it best not to ask.

A few hours later Deanna and I were permitted to enter the PICU room where Zachary was laying. Like we had seen many times, Zachary's condition was not a sight for the faint of heart. He was puffy, fully sedated and had lots of tubes emanating from his body. But from our point of view he looked great. His vital signs were rock solid and his orange-ish glow skin color was now more like Mom & Dad's. The new liver had only been in his body for 8 hours and already it was performing remarkably well.

Blog: Transplant Call

Submitted 4/24/2008

It was about 3am when the phone rang. I struggled to wake up and reach for the phone. Who could this be? No one calls me at 3am unless it is really important. The voice on the other end of the phone was one of the Transplant surgeons at Children's. He informed me that donor organs for Zachary had become available a few states away.

Suddenly I'm wide awake and listening.

I received only a small bit of information about the donor but the important thing was that the size and blood type were a match. The doctor gave me the itinerary for the next few hours and what to expect. Apparently he needed to fly to the hospital where the donor had passed and visually inspect the organs to confirm that they were indeed in good condition. He expected the transplant team to begin prepping Zachary for the Operating Room at around 8am. Get some rest he said. It is going to be a long day.

I've been up since 3am.

So how did this come about? My last journal entry painted a somewhat bleak picture of Zachary's condition. The best explanation is that the little guy simply fought back and improved his health. The problems of blood pressure, breathing issues and high ammonia levels stabilized. Frankly, I have absolutely no idea how he rebounded from such dire straits. Yet he did and his timing couldn't have been more perfect.

I've been nagging Deanna for some time to get out of Dodge. "Go visit your parents in Chardon (Cleveland). Take Aidan with you and relax". For once in a blue moon she actually took my advice and left just yesterday. Ironically, I am now calling her at 3:15am and basically asking her to come back. Looks like she will never take my advice again.

Zachary was taken to the OR at 8am as expected. The doctors will remove his liver, small intestine, stomach, pancreas and perhaps gall bladder. This is a very lengthy surgery that will last approximately 12 plus hours. We anticipate seeing Zachary back in the PICU later this evening probably a little swollen with a case of bed head. It's been a long wait and even though there was a rocky road of health issues along the way we are ready to transition from pre-transplant problems to post-transplant recovery.

Just to remind everyone, post-transplant recovery will still be lengthy - 9 months perhaps. But if all goes well, we can change residency from our digs in Pittsburgh back to our Severna Park (Maryland) house after around 4 months. After everything we have been through these past 10 months or so, this sounds like a pretty good plan.

However, let's not put the cart before the horse just yet. This is a very draining surgery and one that will take a lot of oomph out of him. Zachary still needs all your positive vibes in any and all forms necessary.

Brian & Deanna

Blog: Transplant Update

Submitted 4/24/2008

Deanna and I have been getting updates every two hours from liaisons of the transplant team and/or the lead transplant surgeon himself. Gone are the niceties from normal phone conversations. No chit-chat, just the facts. So far the facts are looking good.

What we know is that the first incision was at 9:30am. Zachary, as expected, had numerous organs removed including the liver, small bowel, stomach, pancreas and gall bladder. From my conversation with the doctor, it looks like the replacement organs, taken from a slightly larger donor, would still be able to fit within Zachary's abdomen. There was some earlier concern that after surgical swelling the doctors would have to resort to some sort of Gortex membrane to act as a temporary skin-like patch. This patch would have been removed when the swelling reduced and Zachary's belly skin could be stretched enough to close the open wound.

Pretty much a mute point actually as this wasn't needed. But hey, if I had to learn this bit of medical knowledge I figured that you, the reader would too.

The liver was a HUGE factor in Zachary's downward trend and deserves some elaboration. In normal people, the liver is like a hunk of...well, like the liver you see at the butcher's shop. It is pink, soft and flexible. According to the transplant surgeon, Zachary's liver looked nothing like this. His liver was so bad that the doctor compared it to an enlarged crusted brick. It certainly needed to go. In fact, the surgeon stated that it was one of the worst livers that he has seen.

And he has seen his fair share of livers.

So as Deanna and I share an empty section of the waiting room we try to pass the time until the next update. This would involve some sort of pacing, nervous foot tapping and numerous unnecessary trips to the bathroom.

We are very appreciative of all of the phone messages, emails and comments on this web site. Zachary's fan base is certainly coast to coast and the amount of support for Deanna and myself has been spectacular.

Yeah, so far this has been a long day but in all honesty we wouldn't have it any other way.

Brian & Deanna

Blog: Which Leads To ...

Submitted 5/15/2008

It's 4pm and I find myself once again occupying a chair in the surgical waiting room. The room is almost at full capacity as I watch a number of people expressing either a blank stare at the tv, looking non-enthusiastically at a Parenting magazine or passing the time downing a few Snicker's candy bars and a Diet Pepsi. Everyone has their own way of dealing with waiting.

Personally I write.

Zachary is currently undergoing brain surgery – or rather a brain procedure as they call it. So how did this come about? How does a 22 month old go from a successful multi organ transplant to brain surgery...ah sorry, a brain procedure, within a few weeks? The story actually began about a week ago. As Zachary's sedation was beginning to be weaned down he began, as expected, to move around. Small movements really but movements never-the-less. At this time Deanna noticed that Zachary was not moving his right leg and brought this to the attention of the PICU attending doctor.

Which leads to ...

A sonogram (ultrasound) was ordered for right leg. It was suspected that maybe a fracture had occurred due to low bone density commonly found with kids who have been bed ridden for this length of time. Perhaps a nerve was being pinched and that this could be the reason for the leg's lack of movements. The sonogram eventually showed both of these theories not to be the case.

Which leads to...

An xray was ordered for the whole right side leg/hip area. The doctors thought that Zachary's hip socket was dislocated during his numerous handlings. The xray showed that Zachary's hip to be a-okay.

Which leads to...

An MRI was ordered for the spine and brain. The thought process here was that maybe the spine had something broken (sorry, not sure of the medical technical term) or that the problem might actually lie somewhere in the brain. The results showed that the spine was fine BUT that a brain abscess (pocket of space) had developed and in all likelihood harbored an infection. I'm told that this infection is in the part of the brain that controls motor skills. Anyone want to guess what part this brain sector controlled? If you guessed the right leg you win the prize.

Which leads to...

The Infectious Disease people were brought in to figure out what kind of infection was causing the ruckus. Even though they had a good idea of the type of bug they weren't about to start giving antibiotics until they were absolutely sure on what they were dealing with.

Which leads to...

A sample of the spinal fluid needed to be collected. Since this is essentially the same fluid that surrounds the brain the doctors needed to do a lumbar puncture (aka spinal tap). This collection of spinal fluids would be cultured for bugs and (if present) would give the doctors a feel for what kind of bacteria was present in the brain. However, the longevity of steroids used for Zachary's treatments has caused inflammation in the spinal tissues which prevent fluids to travel from the brain to the spine. In other words, the lumbar puncture didn't work too well. This meant that another avenue of collecting spinal fluids needed to be performed.

Which leads to...

The next step up from a lumbar puncture is to collect this fluid directly from the area surrounding the brain. The Neurosurgical doctors tell me that they will collect a sample of fluid and monitor the pressure of this fluid. I'm told that this is a simple procedure that is in fact done at the bedside.

Parents of course, are kicked out of the PICU during this time period - even more if they are sarcastic bloggers.

Brian & Deanna

Blog: The Hike Downhill

Submitted 5/13/2008

A few years back Deanna and I hiked up one of the mountains east of Seattle. We were accompanied with good friends who, like us, enjoyed the whole granola-eating-tree-hugging-Birkenstock-wearing lifestyle. The hike up was grueling for sure and required a few breaks to catch our breaths. At the top of the mountain was our reward - a great view which we savored while eating our lunch of hiker-friendly pb&j sandwiches. With the hard part of the hike over we headed down the trail. Oh sure the hike down consisted of the same amount of steps but as we all know, hiking downhill is a whole lot easy than hiking uphill.

As our caravan of four trekkers were making their way down the trail, yours truly stepped into a pothole of sorts and heard my ankle snap (could have been a crackle or a pop). I don't remember the exact sound as I was too busy filling the air with noises of my own. Most of which I can't repeat in this blog. So here we were: four miles from the trail head and I can't stand, can't walk and complaining to anyone who will listen.

As bad as it seemed, I was comforted in knowing that the group all had medical training. Deanna, of course is a physical therapist, and our friend's professions consisted of an occupational therapist and an emergency room doctor. I, of course, used to watch General Hospital while in college. Surely this group could solve my painful woes. Perhaps some sort of special ankle therapy or a magic pill would take away my pain. Their collective advice took a different route: Stay off of the ankle and let the body heal the wound.

Not exactly what I wanted to hear but my friends continued to assist me down the mountain every step of the way.

Zachary's whole life at this point has consisted of an uphill hike. All of the surgical procedures represent the grueling steps up the mountain path. He has fallen down a few times but always managed to take a deep breath, get back up and finish his uphill journey. The transplant is like Zachary's pb&j lunch break. He is still in the adjustment phase of new organs and working out the kinks. It's been a few weeks and now he is starting his hike downhill. It is expected to be just as long as his trip uphill and hopefully will be uneventful. At least that is our wish.

Zachary had his second post transplant surgical procedure last Wednesday. The surgeons were limited on just how far the skin would stretch across the abdomen. In the end they couldn't close it completely and left Zachary with an opening about the size of an orange. The opening is covered with some sort of medical clear duct tape that will eventually be absorbed into the body. In the time being, Zachary's skin will begin to grow into this open area and eventually close the wound on its own. How long this will take is a guess - perhaps a few months give or take a week.

Unfortunately Zachary has recently acquired another infection which is currently being treated with antibiotics. These bugs are proving a little harder to evict than anticipated due to the fact that Zachary is already on a *daily diet of immunosuppressant drugs. The two just don't go together very well.*

His breathing issues are holding steady. Not a whole lot of improvements but then again no backsliding either. The doctors tell me that they could be a little more aggressive but until the wound heals up a little more it is in Zachary's best interest to be on the breathing machine. Be patient they say. There is no magic pill. Let his body heal itself. Now where have I heard this before?

The bottom line is that Zachary was a very sick kid before the transplant. Even though his new organs are working great the fact remains that he is still a sick kid. There are still issues to tackle and hoops to jump through to complete the healing process. It won't all happen today of course but over the next several months we hope that it all works out for the better. It will take time and we'll be there by his side every day.

In the meantime let's hope Zachary doesn't step in any potholes.

Brian & Deanna

Blog: The Math

Submitted 5/06/2008

Back in my college days I took a lot of math classes. Whether it was Calculus, Statistics or general Business courses we were always given some sort of problem to solve. It didn't matter if the problem started with a train leaving Station A at 3 o'clock or if Mr. Smith invested $5,000 at a rate of 6%. The purpose was to solve the problem using pluses, minuses and some sort of algebraic equation.

The key to solving the problems was to take away all of the fluff and focus on the essential facts. In the end it all came down to the math. Eventually you get into the mindset of thinking like a computer and zeroing in on what is important. And if that didn't work you copied the person's work sitting next to you.

Prior to the transplant, solving Zachary's medical problems seemed to involve the same sort of thinking. Station A would be replaced by liver tests. A rate of 6% was now some type of blood test result. The solution involved taking all of the pertinent variables and solving the equation. The doctors would study his lab results in much the same way as I did story problems. In the end they would work out the solution to Zachary's problems – usually without resorting to copying anyone else's work.

Of course it wasn't always easy. Zachary made sure of that. There was always something going on that didn't quite add up and more times than not, the doctors needed a few days to figure it out. It was those few days that seemed to last forever. But I would like to think that that is all in the past now.

Is it okay to think like this?

It's a strange feeling seeing Zachary getting better on a daily basis. Don't get me wrong, we are all for it. It is just that over the past umpteen months we have become accustomed to hearing about a new problem every time we entered the PICU. But since the transplant we have seen nothing but positive changes and significant improvements. That light at the end of the tunnel appears to be closing in on us. It is difficult to fully embrace this new way of thinking but we are starting to come around to it.

Zachary's open wound is healing quite nicely. The scheduled procedure to close it further was pushed back from yesterday to tomorrow. The doctors want a few extra days of healing to allow the swelling to go down even more. So far the intestinal scopes, biopsies and blood tests are showing healthy organs. No signs of rejection yet.

Speaking of rejection, statistically every 6 of 10 transplant patients have some form of rejection. Of those

6, two are considered to have some form of severe rejection. To compensate, any level of rejection requires an appropriate amount of immunosuppressant drugs and steroids. So far Zachary is on both of these drugs to minimize initial signs of rejection. As time goes on, the drug levels will be adjusted accordingly. Either way, the staff is monitoring the situation for any and all signs of problems.

Currently Zachary is still fully sedated, paralyzed and on low ventilator settings. Every day he continues to lose much of the fluid that he gained during surgery and in doing so makes it easy to suture his wound shut. Shortly after the suturing is done the doctors will stop the paralyzing drug, decrease the sedation and in all probability remove the ventilator. I have to admit that it will be nice to hold him again.

In the next few days, weeks and months the doctors will poke and prod Zachary so many times that he will, like the rest of us, hate hospitals. But the treatment is definitively for his own good. The doctors have to monitor the organs for a long time before they will cut the cord and let us leave Pittsburgh. In the meantime we continue to start off our days with liver numbers, intestinal numbers and ventilator settings. Hopefully these numbers will continue to improve and allow Zachary to heal and eventually return to our home in Severna Park, Maryland.

Like I said, it all comes down to the math.

Brian & Deanna

Blog: 1968 Plymouth Satellite
Submitted 6/11/2008

We all have those special times in our lives that we never forget. Whether it is our first kiss, winning an award or your first day at school we tend to keep these *memories fresh and at the top of our memory spreadsheet.*

Like most guys I remember fondly my first car. It was essentially a gift from my Granddad. In exchange for mowing his lawn for the summer he gave me the set of keys to his 1968 Plymouth Satellite. The car was clean, ran good and had a 318 V8 engine (argh argh argh and other manly noises). My granddad didn't even charge me a dime. I guess that money wasn't an issue with him.

So here I am – a 16 year old kid with a mean set of wheels and all I had to do was hang out with my grandparents when the front yard needed mowed. I really got the great end of that deal. I'm not sure just what they were thinking but it was clear that I would never understand the senior citizen thought process.

To bring everyone up to speed, last week Zachary had his ventilator scope replaced with a trach. The thought process here (among many others) is that the trach is less restrictive and thus allows for greater mobility. In other words, it was easier to hold Zachary with this type of device. After waiting a few days of wound healing time we finally got the go ahead this past Monday to hold Zachary. If I told you that it was a great feeling to cradle my son in my arms I would be vastly understating the moment.

Thinking back I guess that it was three months ago when Deanna and I last held Zachary. This time however there have been some very important changes. He is significantly less swollen, void of the color orange and most importantly has new organs. During the hour or so that I held him I can't say that I saw him open his eyes or smile. He didn't move his hands towards me or even wake up for that matter. I can say though, that his heart rate and blood pressure settled down and that he appeared calmer than he did that entire morning. Communication, it seems, it not always definable.

Keep in mind that Zachary is still a little loopy due to all of the sedation drugs still swirling around in his body.

As these drugs eventually get weaned down we hope to see increased activity in his arms and legs. I can say that during these past few weeks we have noticed movements, albeit subtle and small, in Zac's extremities. I'll admit that it's not much but it is a start.

From here on out a new chapter has begun. Deanna and I will continue to hold Zachary and encourage him to move around and thus strengthen his muscles. It doesn't really matter if this type of therapy is done at his crib in the PICU or on the floor at our apartment. What matters most is that we get to move forward with our lives and spend time with our son.

Maybe my granddad was on to something after all.

Brian & Deanna

Blog: Sun Block Factor 400

Submitted 5/17/2008

I've never been a big fan of the beach. It's not that I don't like the view of the ocean or the sound of the waves or even the occasional beach ball that gets pounded towards me but what I have never been able to get comfortable with is the sun. You see, the sun is not my friend and as such I tend to burn very easily. I have a condition that keeps my skin from tanning even under the most optimal conditions. The medical term is lobster-boy-itus. It seems that no matter what kind of skin protectant I use, short of Hellman's mayonnaise, I can expect a red burn just from walking from the car to the beach house.

When Zachary was born he had an orange-ish glow about him that was primarily due from the side effects of the bad liver. Even though his skin color was not normal he possessed a far better tan than I had ever experienced. In fact, it was not beyond my realm of thought to hope that his skin might permanently keep some remnants of this hue for the rest of his life. Maybe this was nature's way of evolving past dad's pasty white skin gene. Perhaps it was in the cards for Zachary to star in the remake of Beach Blanket Bingo.

However, after the transplant I must reevaluate my theories. Zachary's liver is doing so well that his skin has not only cleared all of the pre-transplant hues but his skin is experiencing the same Clorox white look that I possess. In other words, he too will probably require sun block factor 400 when playing beach volleyball.

Sorry Zachary – Hollywood will not be calling.

Brian & Deanna

Blog: Chess Match

Submitted 5/29/2008

I used to play chess in my high school and college days. I didn't win any national championships but I'd like to think that I was somewhere between novice and decent. By most opinions, chess is a game of logic, probability and the ability to predict future conditions. Of course in my case it also included a huge amount of luck. Chess involves the association of all of your pieces (think team sport) and how they interacted with your opponent's pieces.

All of the pieces have their own unique special power for strategical purposes. For instance, the pawn is pretty much a sacrificial piece where as other pieces like the rook, bishop and knight are like the special forces of the chess array. Their purpose essentially is to stealthfully go in and take out their opponent's pieces.

In the world of chess thinking ahead is how you win the game. Timing is everything - hence the strategy and skills of the players.

I see a lot of this type of thought process with Zachary and his medical staff. The doctors are always trying to stay one step ahead of the usual suspects like infections, *fluid over load or sedation levels – basically the hooligans of the post transplant world. The medical staff is doing a great job but like a long lengthy chess match, this takes time.*

Zachary's life will forever be a chess match with no ending. No chance to declare checkmate. This part of his life was dictated since he was three weeks old and diagnosed with NEC (necrotizing enterocolitis). Therefore he will always need follow-up visits with the doctors and will thus incorporate these medical jaunts into his lifestyle. The drive from Severna Park, MD to Pittsburgh is about five hours. More than enough time to teach Zachary the long intricacies of chess. Then again, maybe I'll wait until he is a few years older.

Perhaps we'll start off with a game of checkers.

Brian & Deanna

Blog: Wingman

Submitted 6/03/2008

Right out of high school a friend and I decided to enlist in the Air Force National Guard. I guess we had visions of flying fighter jets around the Lima, Ohio area on weekends. But first we had to prove that we were healthy American manly men. It was a cold winter morning when we drove to the Springfield (Dayton) recruiting office for the grueling physical. We did a few pushups, a few chin ups and then stepped on the scale. Child's play back then but today I would probably require some form oxygen to complete those tasks.

I remember that we rushed through this entire medical process just to wait for the results. "Hurry up and wait" the recruiting guys joked. No problem as it gave us ample time to come up with our cool Top Gun nicknames. Since Maverick and Goose were taken I was leaning towards Caffeine or Latte. Unfortunately, due to my flat feet and not so perfect eye sight I failed the physical. My buddy would have no wingman on his weekend fly-bys around the Lima Mall.

But my brief afternoon with the military taught me one valuable lesson – how to wait.

Zachary's tracheostomy is scheduled for today. Well, "scheduled" is not the best word here. They tell me that Zachary is listed as an add-on patient for this procedure. For those of you new to this medical jargon, "add-on" is surgical code for "we'll try to fit you in if we have the time".

It is essentially comparable to walking in to the hair salon and trying to snag a trim without an appointment. Thus we are at the mercy of open surgical time slots. In the meantime I will remain with my new wingman until the surgical doctors arrive to wheel Zachary away.

Brian & Deanna

Blog: The Glass Door Incident

Never Submitted

Hospitals and me really never developed that buddy-buddy warm and fuzzy feeling. More like an uneasy alliance whenever an emergency came up. It's not like I've never been to a hospital. In fact I started my life in one. But throughout my time here on Earth I, like most people, tend to stay clear of this environment. One of the few times that I was a patient in an Emergency Room revolved around a series of comical errors and bad timing decisions – essentially setting the stage for my opinion on emergency room venues. Since it is important to laugh at one's endeavors I will provide the play by play.

The time was college. Like many of my friends I was several pounds lighter and in better physical shape. I jogged every day and followed up with the standard testosterone regime of push ups, chip ups and sit ups.

And no matter what I ate – whether it be greasy potato chips, fatty hamburgers or double scoop chocolate fudge ice cream with extra sprinkles I could work it off by running a lap or two (or three) around the campus. Now that I look back on it, life was kinda easy.

One day I was running through the campus of Ohio State University. It was one of those days where the sky was sunny, the temperature was comfortable and a slight breeze was on my face. The bad side of this scenario was that I just happened to be hitting my peak stride on the sidewalk around some of the shops on the main drag called High Street. This sidewalk happened to harbor several large doors...several large glass doors...several large glass doors that swung OUT onto the sidewalk. During this stretch of my exercise program I noticed that I had better pick up the pace somewhat or I would miss the green light about a hundred yards up the street. From past experience I knew that missing this light would cause me several minutes of downtime.

Missing the light was not an option.

So I went from a fast jog to a fast sprint. As I stared at the light (and the pretty coed walking across the street) I sorta took my eyes off of the sidewalk. Somewhere between staring at the sidewalk, the light and the coed I missed the open swinging glass door emanating from the hair salon. And as quickly as I decided to pick up the pace a large sheet of glass decided otherwise. Enter the term "Rapid Deceleration".

The end result was a broken glass door and a jogger laying comatose nearby with a bloody face and pieces of glass embedded in my forehead, forearms and knees. My next memory was of several beauticians standing over me trying to figure out if I was dead or alive. Not exactly my proudest moment.

However embarrassing this moment was, it paled to what was in store for me later. As I sat on the hospital bed in the Emergency Room I had to explain this story to a doctor who, to his credit, maintained a straight face throughout my entire story. The nurses though, were not so elegant. One after another came in with a clipboard asking me questions about the incident. One after another left my waiting area only to whisper their findings to their group of coworkers whereas another medical groupie would emerge to ask me a slightly different version of the same question.

So it stands to reason that I was emotionally scarred by this hospital trauma. Consider me a victim of some crazily misunderstood athletic accident. In spite of the amount of time that has gone by since that summer day in 1985 but I still think about it when I enter the hospital. In all probability I will remind this to Zachary often when he gets older. Although I suspect that my son will have developed his own story by then.

Probably far better than mine.

Brian & Deanna

Blog: 2nd Year Birthday Party, by Deanna
Submitted 7/02/2008

It's been two years since the boys were born on July 2nd. What an emotional two years it has been. Brian and I were thinking back to their actually delivery date. It was around midnight on July 1st that my water broke. I woke Brian up and I don't think that he really believed me. I couldn't believe it myself... it was too early I kept saying. I was only 32 weeks. We hadn't even painted the nursery or set up the cribs yet!

I called the doctor and he advised us to come into the hospital right away. I took a shower and Brian's mom packed him a lunch and made coffee. Luckily, his parents were visiting at the time in order to watch the dog and cat for us. We made the 45 minute drive to Greater Baltimore Medical Center in record time. Not a lot of traffic on the road at that hour. I was feeling fine and only experiencing mild back pain (possible contractions?). When we arrived they hooked me up to the fetal monitors and I laid back to hear the beautiful sound of the boys heart beat. All would be fine I kept telling myself.

Then we were told that there were no beds in the NICU and that we would need to transfer to another hospital. "Where did we want to go?", the nurse asked. We hadn't even considered this possibility and being new to Baltimore, we had no clue where else to go. They suggested a few hospitals, but after making several phone calls we were told that only the University of Maryland had "room at the inn". I was transported via ambulance to this new destination while Brian tried to follow in our car.

By the time we arrived there was no stopping the delivery and since the boys were both breech, I was scheduled for a C-section. Aidan was born at 12:16pm and Zachary 12:18pm on July 2, 2006. I was excited to hear their cries upon delivery and Brian got to hold them both. They were whisked away to the NICU for testing. The next morning we were able to spend some quality time with the boys and it appeared that all was fine. How naïve I was back then! The "honeymoon" was over at 3 weeks when we were told that Zac was diagnosed with necrotizing enterocolitis and rushed into emergency surgery. He survived his first surgery and has been fighting ever since.

Today we brought Aidan into the PICU to visit Zac. They haven't seen each other since February. As soon as Zac saw Aidan he got the biggest smile on his face. He hadn't smiled for Mom and Dad yet, but for his brother he was all smiles. Then the nursing staff sang "Happy Birthday" to the boys and it just brought tears to my eyes. We didn't know if Zac would see his 2nd birthday, but here we were with the whole family together.

Thanks to my parents (Bob and Chris Joss), Ann & Peg Korecko, and Jill & Ally Heinz for joining in the boys' birthday celebration today. We appreciate all the emails and phone calls as well. It has been a wonderful day and I am so proud of my boys.

Happy Birthday Aidan and Zachary... Love, Mom.

Blog: *Columbus Marathon*

Submitted 7/08/2008

The other morning I was running late and had to sacrifice my "coffee to go" mug. Ever notice that no one riding the bus wants to share a seat with a strange man who has the jitters? Upon arrival to Childrens I first swung by the small PICU waiting room – the one with the free coffee and extremely small cups. Sometimes you have to compromise your values.

Unbeknownst to me there is an understanding amongst some coffee drinking humans that it is socially acceptable to begin verbal conversations with other coffee drinking humans during the early morning fill up stage. Normally this is not a bad thing but it probably would be best if this exchange of words comes after...way after the first cup of coffee is consumed by both parties.

This particular gentleman (who, btw was on his 2nd cup of joe) said that he had saw me around the PICU and inquired about my son's status. As I questioned my newly ordained celebrity status as "Zac's Dad" I told him about my son's bout with NEC and the much appreciated multi-organ transplant. In between my gulps of a semi-hot beverage he had to tell me that .... . (sorry but I didn't pay much attention here) and...... (or again here due to the caffeine not kicking in) and.... (still hasn't kicked in)...and then he stated that Zac was in a marathon and not a sprint.

Yes I've heard this phrase mentioned more than a dozen times over the past two years. And yes I must admit that it is as true this time as it was the first time or any other time for that matter when I heard it. Everyone would agree that marathons are long and arduous and also important to personally add is that they are not especially fun or graceful.

I've run one marathon in my life. The course was a 26 mile race through the streets of Columbus, Ohio. It was a chilly November morning back in 1988 when a few of my friends decided to embark on this memorable journey. Somewhere during the 15th mile marker I really questioned why we decided on this absurd adventure. What were we trying to prove?

My memories of the race are not especially worth bragging about. I hit the wall at the 18th mile. I was passed up by not one but two blind men. A lady with a shirt on that said "Go For It Grandma" whizzed by me. Finally, there was that group of four white haired ladies who passed me up discussing cooking utensils the entire way.

The final segment of the race was long straight shot of pavement that gave the runners an unimpeded view of the home stretch.   The good news is that I could see just how far I needed to jog to finish. The bad news is that could see just how far I needed to jog to finish. At times I felt like I was running on a treadmill never making ground. In order to keep some aspect of motivation I had to focus on the small stuff. Keep going until the end of the block. Keep going until the light. Keep going until you past the live band (yes there was a live band). Eventually I kept at it and finally crossed the finish line.

I was tired and worn out and in all probability didn't gain any style points on my final kick. Still, I was very happy of my accomplishment.

Zachary is past the treadmill part and now on his final stretch of his marathon. Like my race, he is focusing on small increments of improvements. The amount of drugs once necessary for his survival has been reduced dramatically. His high level of sedation, once imperative to his comfort is now so low that it is only a matter of a few weeks before it is totally gone. His ventilator, once considered an external organ has such low settings that the respiratory therapists are discussing how to transition to a portable home unit for supplemental support.

Months ago the doctors would hang out at Zac's crib during rounds and discuss his problems – taking a very long time in doing so. Not a very uplifting experience. Now their pit stop at Zachary's crib is more like a brief commercial break. The atmosphere is not stressful but full of optimism and confidence.

As parents we hold him daily and watch him focus his eyes on our faces as well as the Elmo balloon swaying in his crib. We were told that when his sedation was reduced that he would move more each day. The docs were on the money there. Smiles are still a rarity but we feel that they will soon be coming on strong. Discharge is inevitable.

Several years down the road Zac may want to run his own marathon...for fun of course. He certainly has nothing to prove to anyone.

Brian & Deanna

Blog: Sisyphus

Submitted 8/05/2008

According to Greek mythology, Sisyphus was sentenced to eternity in Hades to perform the same task over and over again. The former King of Corinth was forced to exert all of his physical might just to roll a huge boulder up a hill. However, just before he reached the summit the darn rock would roll back down the hill again. As frustrating as it was, this was the punishment that Sisyphus had to endure. Again and again and again.

Sisyphus probably thought that he had it bad. Eh, maybe he did. But in all probability he wouldn't have complained so much if he had to ride the city bus to Children's every day and eat at the hospital cafeteria.

After a lengthy wait, Zachary finally got his 4th MRI to determine if the brain abscesses that he developed weeks ago diminished. If you remember, Zachary had developed small lesions in a few different areas of his brain. After 3 different MRI's showed nonspecific behavior (growth) it was suggested that a noninvasive approach should continue to be utilized. Thus Zachary was kept on some pretty hefty amounts of antibiotics and antifungal medicines in hope of decreasing these abscesses.

As it turns out the latest MRI showed no such luck in any such progress. The abscesses didn't recede at all but on the plus side they didn't increase in size either. So after weeks of injecting Zachary with antibiotics and antifungal medicine in hopes of curing the brain lesions, this all appears to have been in vain. Of course, one could argue that the absence of any growth was attributed to these very medicines. This, of course, is like arguing that carrying a lucky penny keeps away blue elephants. It is hard to disprove what you can't see.

We are, it seems, at a crossroad. One option is to stay the course and continue to bombard Zachary with the same antibiotic/antifungal medicines. Perhaps with this route the lesions will eventually disappear. Perhaps we just need to be patient and wait for results. The other option is to be a little more aggressive and obtain yet another biopsy. The theory here is that if some brain matter is retrieved then the doctors can actually see just what they are combating and use only one medicine. Of course it is entirely possible that there is nothing to retrieve and that the lesions are filled up with a whole lot of empty. Sorta like a hole in the ground – nothing but space.

We are straddling the fence on this decision at the moment. Zachary has traveled down the biopsy path before which yielded no results. The reasons for this proposed biopsy is still to determine the cause of the lesions. The surgeon tells us that this avenue of entry into the brain has changed somewhat and thus poses less risk. Of course, anytime you shove a needle into the brain you are accepting a certain amount of risk.

Sigh. We are so close to discharge that it pains us to watch this rock roll down the hill another time. Once more, there is an issue standing in the way of Zachary's journey back home. Yet as parents we continue to push the boulder up the hill once again. Hopefully this will be the last time.

Brian & Deanna

Chapter 20

Beyond Children's Hospital

few days after the transplant surgery Zachary's recovery was right on target. His swelling had begun to subside, his medications were lessened and all of his blood tests pointed to a very healthy patient. In general Zachary was doing everything that the doctors wanted. He was healing up quite nicely.

It wasn't long before we started to introduce the term "Discharge" with the transplant doctors. At first it was a rather nonchalant reference at the end of a statement. Then as the days passed the term was moved up a notch to the middle of the sentence and then finally it became the lead off word in our opening dialogues... MANY of our opening dialogues.

To their credit, the transplant doctors were very good about using the politician speech – that it, talking a lot about discharge but not really answering the question of when. I suppose that from their side of the fence there were many other possible issues to content with and discharge was not a topic to be considered at that time.

In all fairness to our parental curiosity, we were not looking for an exact day for discharge. That would be rather unfair and totally unrealistic. We were understanding parents and would have been satisfied with a range of say,

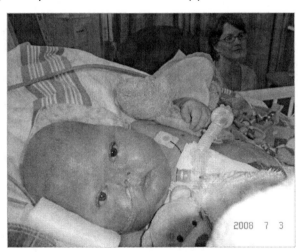

Zachary with Deanna in background

three days. Is that not too much to ask? After all, even the cable guy can give us a four-hour window for his service.

We soon learned that there are many reasons why the term discharge was not mentioned. Here are a few:

Infections

On May 29, 2008 - almost a month past his transplant Zachary became infected with not one but three different bugs. Of course, all three bugs needed their own distinct antibiotics in the process which only compounded his fluid overload problem. These bugs set Zac back in virtually all areas of improvement ranging from ventilator settings, rejection issues, enteral (belly) feedings and fluid gain. It took a few weeks but his body fought off the infections, which allowed the doctors to resume his recovery process.

GVHD

On June 21, 2008 Zachary's skin started to look red and blotchy. We were not sure if this was a reaction to his enteral feeds or perhaps some sort of post transplant rash. After a few days had passed a skin biopsy was performed and the results were devastating. Zachary has developed GVHD (Graft vs. Host Disease).

GVHD is essentially a turf war between the new organs and the host body - sorta like the opposite of rejection. In other words, when rejection occurs the body treats the new organs as some sort of invading party and sends out it's squadron of attack cells for combat. In GVHD, it is the new organs that go on the offensive and attack the host body.

From what I could gather from my attempts at internet surfing there are four levels of GVHD ranging from mild irritation to a very bad outcome. The transplant doctor told me that in Zachary's case this level is hovering between three and four – that would be the bad side of the range. Talk about getting the wind knocked out of you.

The longer we waited to combat this disease the worse Zachary's chances would become. The doctors needed to move quickly as time was now our enemy. They immediately lowered Zachary's immunosuppressant drugs along with giving Zachary higher levels of steroids and then waited. It was a stressy week watching from the sidelines but after seven days we saw the rash disappear.

As dangerous as GVHD is to the body, there is some potential for a positive spin. Statistically, when a transplant recipient successfully fights off this disease they greatly lower their chances of rejection in the future. In a way, this turf war demonstrates the new organ's strength within the body. Strong organs, it seems, allow for more stability within the body as a whole.

I guess the saying "what doesn't kill you only makes you stronger" actually applies with organs as well.

Brain Lesions

Long-term exposure to antibiotics tends to promote fungus growth within the body. It's like this: Your body naturally possesses and uses all kinds of bacteria within your body. We will call this "good bacteria". Sometimes your body is invaded by certain bugs that have no business being there and makes the body sick. We will call this "bad bacteria". Many sick patients, like Zachary, have many of these "bad bacteria" which is not effectively killed off by the body's own immune system. So to compensate, the doctors introduce various antibiotics designed to kill off the "bad bacteria". The problem is that these antibiotics treat "bad bacteria" and "good bacteria" the same way and tend to kill them both off.

Without good bacteria occupying space, other organisms tend to move in including fungi. When this particular organism enters the body it becomes very difficult to eradicate. It is hard enough to kill fungus when it is in the chest cavity – harder still when it invades the brain. Still even harder when the patient is immunosuppressed like Zachary.

Some time after Zachary's transplant a MRI showed the development of certain lesions (non definable space) within the brain. Lesions within the brain could and most often do pose devastating problems for the brain. Areas such as motor skills, hearing, and intelligence could all be compromising by-products of brain lesions. Left unchecked, these lesions could grow and compound the problem to dangerous levels including death. The doctors gave Zachary a 25% chance of overcoming this issue.

The problem is that no one really could say with absolute certainty that these lesions were a result of a fungus, bacteria or a cancerous tumor. Unfortunately we had only a few limited options.

1. Zachary could be treated for an unknown span of time with a hodge-podge of antibiotics and/or antifungal medicines. Then he would undergo routine MRIs in order to monitor progression.
2. The second option is to do a brain biopsy. Provided that the actual act of inserting a needle into Zac's brain doesn't do more damage than it solves.
3. There was no third option.

There was no up-to-date road map to follow here. No exact list of ingredients to follow in eradicating the brain lesions. In fact, no one really knew just what we were combating. It was like we were shooting in the dark. The Infectious Disease folks were trying to make these lesions go away with their best possible guess of antibiotic and antifungal medicines. The game plan here was to inundate Zachary with these drugs in hope that it will take care of the lesions.

After several snapshots at Zachary's brain with MRI (Magnetic Resonance Imagery) technology it became apparent that the lesions were just not going away. In fact, there was some disagreement amongst the staff on whether they were growing or getting smaller. In the case of a tie, it seems, the parent gets to make the deciding vote. So with a lot of thought, Deanna and I decided that knowing what was in Zachary's brain was better than not knowing what was in Zachary's brain. Hence we opted for the biopsy.

Thankfully it was the correct decision as the surgery went off without incident. The neurosurgeon who performed the surgery told us that she retrieved remnants of a fungus encapsulated within a clump of dead cells. This fungus, as it turns out was very hard to detect and even harder to treat. Still, we now had an antifungal plan of attack that was more strategic and precise.

This long-term method was to take place over the next several months. If all went well there would be nothing left but some dead clusters of fungus cells located deep within his brain and a nasty scar on the side of his head. Hopefully Zachary will develop a great story to go along with the scar.

As the months passed Zachary's clinical appearance and the way that he acted generally seemed quite positive. His motor skills were advancing and his mental acuity seemed to improve. The real barometer of success was the subsequent MRI's which showed a reduction in the size of the lesions. It appears that Zachary was once again beating the odds.

On July 22, 2008 just three months since his transplant surgery Zachary was deemed healthy enough to leave the PICU. It was a momentous day for sure but one that passed without any fanfare or celebration. The process was simple. Zachary was wheeled out of the PICU to the step down unit referred to as 7 South. Some medical sheets were handled off and a handshake was given. The nurses went back to their jobs and Zachary was officially one step closer to discharge.

Shortly after Zachary starting occupying his new digs at 7 South all of the medical power players started talking with a different slang. Of course, everyone from the transplant doctors to the janitorial staff knew that Zachary was healthy enough to leave the protective arm of Children's Hospital. At this point, the medical staff started using phrases like "leaving 7 South" and "exiting the hospital" in their conversations with us. They talked with a sense of closure in each sentence. Suddenly there was a new feeling in the air. Discharge was on the tip of everyone's tongue.

On Tuesday August 25, 2008, after being hospitalized for nearly one full year, Zachary Mason Johnson was officially discharged from Children's Hospital of Pittsburgh.

Blog: Madeline Kate Johnson

Submitted 8/15/2008

Yesterday at around 2:30pm Deanna gave birth to a beautiful healthy baby girl.

Weight: 7 lb 2 oz

Height: 18 ½ inches

Name: Madeline (Maddie) Kate

Thursday morning at 1am I was notified by Deanna that her water had broke. Now, at this time I am considering myself a seasoned veteran of the late night important news saga. You see, two years ago when the twins were announcing their arrival plans I went through this very scenario. Back then I was in panic mode and really didn't perform in a calm manner. Since then I have had time to perfect this art and now feel that I was completely ready for the occasion.

So Thursday morning I calmly got out of bed and proceeded to get things together for the trip to the hospital. Clothes for the mom-to-be were packed by Deanna the prior week. The directions to West Penn Hospital were jotted down on memo pad by Deanna. Finally, my parents were awakened from their sleep in anticipation of some last minute instructions on Aidan's schedule by Deanna. Obviously I was doing a great job.

Upon arrival to the hospital I embraced my newly developed role as pack mule and carried in the luggage through the entrance doors behind my still very pregnant wife. Throughout it all I managed to forget my toiletries and ended up using the hospital supplied tooth brush (definately not ADA approved). Maybe my wife should have been in charge of packing my gear as well.

Deanna is still feeling a little tired but nevertheless just fine. We anticipate leaving the hospital with little Maddie and adjusting to a life in our apartment until the next week when Zachary is discharged. Yes, our lives certainly do not parallel anything stagnant or boring.

Brian & Deanna

Chapter 21

The Children's Home

Although we had hoped to have Zachary discharged to our home in Maryland, the transplant doctors weren't quite ready to have our son that far away just that soon. For their comfort level, they proposed discharging Zac to our apartment in nearby Shadyside (Pittsburgh) for the next three months. With a semblance of a normal family life coupled with the close proximity to Children's Hospital this seemed to be a reasonable compromise for the next few months.

Of course this plan was doomed from the beginning as Maryland Medicaid balked of the idea of paying for nursing care outside of the State of Maryland. Apparently, the purse strings of this 800-pound gorilla trumped our most reasonable plan for Zachary's recovery.

So a Plan B needed to be developed.

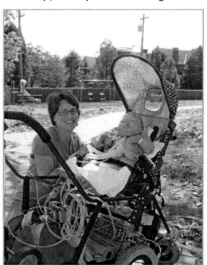

The alternative idea was to have Zachary discharged to a local hospital like environment called The Children's Home. This facility is a hybrid of hospital and home and was created to help educate parents in the various medical methods needed to care for their sick children. This additional training helped to facilitate a more successful discharge to a home environment.

The Children's Home has a round the clock nursing staff

Deanna & Zac at TCH

combined with many of the comforts of a home environment like a kitchen, family room and playroom. It wasn't the living room of the Waltons but it was nice to have the whole family in one room.

As it turns out, this was an ideal transition from the PICU of Children's Hospital to our ranch home in Maryland. The staff furthered our training in fine tuning our nursing skills regarding Zachary's medicines, his home ventilator and trach. Plus it helped us to get around the 800-pound gorilla.

From a simple internet search one can find a Children's Home in cities ranging from Tampa, Winston-Salem, Catonsville (Baltimore) and Cincinnati to name a few. I can't speak for these other locations but I'm told that the Pittsburgh location is unique in its overall purpose. The common trait of a name is about as far as similarities go with this facility.

The bottom line is that The Children's Home is a lot like the fish parable. Instead of giving sushi to anyone walking down the street you teach them to fish...or something of that nature. With this extremely horrible analogy, the parents are taught how to care for their children and not rely on a nursing staff as a long term crutch. The premise of educating parents on the intricacies of childcare turned out to be a smart idea.

It didn't take long for Deanna and I to become quite comfortable with giving the large amounts of medicines and other types of daily care to Zachary. What once was perceived as an overwhelming amount of work at the PICU quickly became a confident routine day in and day out at The Children's Home. The nurses at this new facility did a great job of making this possible.

Leading up to the final days of our stay in Pittsburgh we started making preparations for our trip home. Deanna began the task of packing up our belongings. She got our mail forwarded as well as coordinated the hookup of Internet and cablevision to our house. Deanna was to leave Pittsburgh with Aidan and Maddie a week ahead of me in order to get the house settled in anticipation of Zachary's arrival. My role was to clean out the apartment and fly back with Zachary when the time came.

Of course we all know that nothing ever goes the way you want it. This is especially true with Zachary Johnson. On Friday October 17, 2008 – just a few days before our planned discharge Zachary developed a line infection. To elaborate a little here, a line infection indicates that a bug could be colonizing on the plastic line located in the blood vessel or worse, it could be brewing in the circulatory system itself. This type of infection could have very serious life altering consequences and needed to be addressed immediately. So the trip back to Children's, no matter what the duration, received little resistance from either Deanna or myself.

The end result was that this round of infection eviction took a week to clear up and made Zachary as good as new. He was then transported back to The Children's Home for another week (or more) of observation and preparation for his trip home to Severna Park, Maryland.

Deanna and I had to accept that this last minute return trip to Children's Hospital was perhaps an omen of things to come. In all probability these trips will be commonplace in the future and in all likelihood happen in the middle of the night, on weekends or on a holiday. Basically a lot like the conditions that we experienced upon his call for organs. The world of transplant recipients adheres to no clock.

The word "normal" will never fully or accurately describe our household life. From here on out we will simply follow a family schedule of unpredictability, chaos and a black hole of unknowns – basically a lot like most every other family in today's world. It looks like the Johnson's will fit in just fine after all.

On Wednesday, November 5, 2008 Zachary Mason Johnson was officially discharged from The Children's Home.

Blog: Pods

Submitted 9/29/2008

As an unknown date for discharge looms somewhere out on the horizon, Deanna and I have begun the process of preparing for the move back to Maryland. My wife will leave Pittsburgh at the end of this week in order to get the house ready for a family of five. Although my Y chromosome doesn't fully understand what this entails I suspect that it means stocking up on paper products, mopping the floors and vacuuming the dust bunnies from under the couch.

Moving our belongings from the apartment to the house is also slated for later this week. Looking back when we first moved into our apartment the plan was simply to live there. The word "nesting" was never mentioned. We were not to buy anything of bulk that would require any heavy lifting or potential moving. We would live like nomads and upon our move out we planned to box up a few things, pack our clothes in some boxes and drive away.

That plan was trashed a few weeks after our move in date. Since we have managed to accumulate various items of bulk within our apartment we have decided to arrange for the use of moving pods. These pods (notice the "s" on the end of the word "pod") are scheduled to be delivered in a few days and will be packed full of accumulated furniture, boxes of toys and kitchen equipment.

I will stick around the Pittsburgh area until Zachary is flown to Maryland within the next week. When next week? Not sure really. This date is kinda hard to pin down as there are various factors that contribute to our departure like written doctor orders, insurance paperwork and nurse staffing.

From what I can tell, most of the "t's" have been crossed and "i's" have been dotted so we should be good to go real soon. If I had to guess on a date I would

anticipate a week or less - give or take a few days for
Zachary to be driven to the airport and boarded up on the
plane.
    I wonder what on-flight movie will be showing?

Brian & Deanna

Blog: Dejohnsonfication
Submitted 10/08/2008
    The bags were packed.
    The kitchen cleaned out.
    The moving boxes were filled and taped shut.
    Our home of the past 13 months has been
Dejohnsonficated.
    Now all that was needed was the back breaking task of
moving the Johnson's accumulated belongings down eight
flights of stairs and past two sets of glass doors to the
moving pods located in the parking lot of the apartment
complex. This labor task force was made up of the
following people:
    Brian. That is all.
    Okay so maybe I exagerrated a little as Deanna did
most of the packing.   I used the elevator and perhaps had
a few hands helping me in the process but at the end of
the day I was still pretty tired. The moving pods are
certainly a great way of transporting one's belongings
from Point A to Point B. The only problem is guessing just
how many pods you actually need. In our circumstance,
we needed 1 1/8 pods. We certainly had enough stuff to
pack into one pod but just a few boxes in the other.
Apparently the pod industry doesn't provide half sizes like
the shoe industry.
    So here is where we stand. Deanna is now back in our
house in Severna Park, MD with both Aidan and Maddie
(and of course her parental labor task force Chris & Bob).
The pods have arrived at their terminal in Maryland and

awaiting the final destination to our house. Deanna will have the much easier job of unpacking the pods (note: no elevator, no glass doors) and putting all of our stuff away. I, on the other hand, have the fun job of hanging with Zachary until he is officially discharged and flown to BWI. In the interim I will work up a sweat by cleaning the apartment, turning in the keys and finishing the kitchen cupboard's last box of macroni and cheese.

We haven't quite closed the book on our time in Pittsburgh but it probably fair to say that we are on the final pages of the last chapter. Zachary's date of discharge is still a moving target but certainly one that is closing in on us. These days of Pittsburgh living are numbered. The end of this era is coming to a close.

Deanna and I appreciate all of your interest and support for Zachary's journey and look forward to a day when this is all a distant memory in our rear view mirror.

Brian & Deanna

Blog: Halloween Gourds

Submitted 10/17/2008

I remember watching the Macy's Thanksgiving Day parade on tv with my dad when I was a kid. Throughout the parade the announcers would always bring up the fact that Santa Claus would soon be upon us. That kept me glued to the tv. Of course, Santa's position in the parade was like the caboose on the train - always destined to be last. In order to catch the main attraction I had to sit through all of the other stuff like the singers, dancers as well as all the Snoopy and Underdog balloons.

After two agonizing hours of sitting through the fluffy stuff the moment was upon me. Finally the big guy himself. Santa Claus was on center stage. I was at the edge of my seat. Upon Saint Nick's arrival the cameras would show the jolly guy surrounded by lots of elfin type people prancing around in green tights. I was about to be dazzled. But based on Santa's stature, he was way past the prancing phase of his life and thus managed only a wave from his sled and then it was over. The credits began to roll.

Only a wave?
No flying reindeer?
No magical toys?
I sat through all of those commercials for this?
I felt jipped.

Waiting for discharge from The Children's Home is on par with sitting through the commercials. At first we were waiting for the home health nurses to get on board with Zachary's schedule. Thankfully that part is behind us. Check. Then we were waiting the Children's Transplant team to coordinate all of Zachary's medical information with their Johns Hopkins counterparts. Again, that part is done. Check. Transportation from PA to MD? Done. Check.

Like the parade, the fluff in Zachary's discharge plan is over. The big event was soon upon us. Monday was marked as the day Zachary would be discharged. We were ready to leave The Children's Home and hang out with the rest of his family, our dog and our home. Monday was not just a penciled in suggested date. It was marked in ink...and red ink at that! The future was soon upon us and history was waiting to be recorded. I was giddy with excitement.

Buuuuuuuuut...(you probably saw this coming)

For some unknown reason, one of the Maryland medical supply vendors backed out from their commitment. This abrupt change forced us to scramble for a Plan B supply company which in turn set our discharge date back a few days (or more). Granted, a few extra days of time in Pittsburgh isn't alot when you consider that we have already been here for 14 months but that's not the point. I'd really like to find this company's knucklehead employee who made this decision and pelt him/her with a large assortment of Halloween gourds found at the local grocery store.

Enough venting. Now on to something less organic.

Lately I've noticed that Zachary is gradually losing the "fat face" often associated with post transplant steroids. Other signs of growth are appearing as well, like a resurgence of hair growth and the addition of more teeth. Zac even has a new set of hearing aids that are allowing him to listen Thomas the Train videos as well as the Chuck Norris movie marathon on Spike TV – consider this the beginning stages of father-son male bonding.

Zachary's quality of hearing is still subject to a best guess. Until he is able to sit in a sound proof booth and raise his hand when he hears a high pitch noise Deanna and I will have to play close attention to his present day body language for signs of his hearing ability. All in all, he continues to make great strides of improvement here at The Children's Home.

So if we have to wait for a later discharge date we will past the time by taking a few more walks outside and watching a few more hours of television inside. In the meantime I'll round up some more gourds.

Brian & Deanna

Blog: The Fish Hook Story

Submitted 10/21/2008

I have buddy in Rhode Island who makes routine trips to the local Emergency Room. It seems that his 11 year old son is quite the athlete and thus tends to push the boundaries of the human body a little more each day. Perhaps a little too much at times. It is not uncommon to find my friend driving to the hospital to deal with his son's issues of broken bones, stitches or even a fish hook stuck in his head.

In all fairness to the fish hook story, I'm told that he still managed to catch a nice sized fish although I'm not quite sure how to visualize that. Apparently this trait (the broken bones, not the fish hook) is common in active kids and although I can't remember it myself, I was reminded by my mother that I too acquired some frequent flyer miles at the local Ohio hospital. These events, of course, are lost in my sea of youth; apparently blocked out by a brain barrier of sorts. Selective memory is a wonderful thing.

As Deanna and I were making plans for our return to Maryland one of the transplant doctors made an odd off-the-cuff comment to me. He said that Zachary will return back to the Children's PICU at a later date. It is not a question of if, but of when. He said that all of the transplant patients return for one reason or another - whether it is an organ rejection issue, an infection or blood test irregularity. The comment was made with such indifference that he barely broke stride while sipping his hot coffee.

His prediction came true last Friday.

That afternoon, just a few days before our discharge from The Children's Home Zachary spiked a small temperature. The usual first wave of remedies was ushered to the front line. A fan usually does the trick. Tylenol was next in line. Neither option worked. A few hours later his temperature showed another slight increase. Later that afternoon his temperature increased even more.

At this point the nurse drew blood samples to determine if an infection was brewing. Within 24 hours we got the bad news. The culture was positive – Zachary had a bug. The obvious decision was made to transport Zac from The Children's Home to the PICU at Children's Hospital for closer observation and antibiotics. The very place that we were fighting like hell to escape from a

month earlier has now become our sanctuary. Ironic isn't
it?

It's been a few days now since the initiation of
antibiotics and it appears that Zachary is doing just fine.
The absence of a fever or low blood pressure suggests
that the bug was contained to the intravenous line and not
running rampant throughout his blood stream. Zachary is
currently resting in his crib, unaware of the close call that
he experienced.

Like my buddy in Rhode Island, the Johnson family has
to accept the fact that we will visit the hospital several
times each year. Aidan may require a cast. Maddie may
need a stitch or two and Zachary will most probably need
further doses of antibiotics.

However, let's hope my kids stay away from the fish
hooks.

Brian & Deanna

Blog: *Thousands of Footprints*

Submitted 11/04/2008

I hear the election results blaring from a tv located in a
common room about 20 feet from this computer. Even
though this election night is an important night for people
all over America the only person that I'm concerned about
at this moment is my son Zachary. He is spending his last
night at The Children's Home in a warm bed surrounded
by monitors that glow and machines that ring. His last
night here will be just like his first. The nursing care will
be constant. Their attention to his needs will be no
different than the night before. Zachary will, by all
accounts, never know the difference.

But even though the routine is the same, everyone
knows that this is not just any normal night. It is
Zachary's last night in Pittsburgh. It is a special night to
be savored in the same way a young child savors

Christmas Eve with the anticipation of presents the next day. Although it is getting late for me too, sleep will have to wait. For now, I am too edgy thinking of what lies in store for my family tomorrow.

Wednesday is Discharge Day for my son. This is the day that we have been looking forward to for a very very long time. The plan is for the ambulance to pick Zachary up at 10am and take him to Allegheny County airport. From there he will board a medical plane that will fly him to Baltimore-Washington International Airport where an ambulance will take him on his final leg to his home in Severna Park, Maryland. Arrival time is somewhere around 1pm.

I've been asked numerous times if I am excited about tomorrow. To be honest I am somewhat calm about the whole thing. Perhaps when the plane is taxing down the runway I'll start hyperventilating with excitement. I can say with 100% conviction that I look forward to returning home to see Deanna, Aidan, Maddie and my dog Bailey. I am looking forward to walking around in my house in my socks, seeing familiar photos on the wall and of course, sleeping in my own bed. Watching Zachary sit on the floor with the rest of the family milling about is what I have been visualizing for months now. These moments are just within my reach.

What my family has gone through over these past several months has been daunting for sure. We have put our lives on a slow motion pace while the rest of the world kept moving forward at regular speed. Even though we endured this gauntlet we know that we didn't do it alone. Many friends, acquaintances and even strangers have helped us along the way. This was a journey that left behind thousands of footprints on our path.

Tomorrow will certainly be a special day for my family, our friends and everyone else who has followed Zachary story over these past two years. But this story doesn't stop here. It will continue for many years to come. Maybe it will be my son's name blaring from a tv set on Election Day years from now. The world is a large place with plenty of opportunities and Zachary is just getting started.

Brian & Deanna

Chapter 22

C l o s u r e

W e knew that we wouldn't get Zachary out of the hospital unscathed. Since he was essentially lying on his back for most of his two years, Zachary was bound to have delayed mental and physical developments. If this wasn't enough, prolonged antibiotics, infections, and repeated uses of diuretics have caused severe hearing loss.

It seems like a lot of negative issues to get angry about, but the bottom line is that our son came home. Not every parent can say that. The problems that Zachary inherited from his initial bout with NEC will certainly stay with him well into adulthood and beyond.

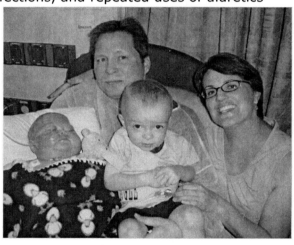

The twin's 2nd birthday from the PICU

Zachary will require physical therapy for his delayed motor skills. He will need creative types of mental stimulation to get him caught up on his IQ levels. As far as his hearing loss goes, there are specialists to consult with on this type of thing.

Throughout this two-year saga our lives continued to evolve. Zachary had loving parents by his side each and every day. Aidan learned to crawl, to walk, and just recently began to jump on the couch, the bed and anywhere else that provided this form of entertainment. During our time in Pittsburgh Deanna became pregnant and just a week before Zachary's discharge from Children's Hospital gave birth to a beautiful baby girl that we named Madeline.

Life, it seems, will always continue to move forward.

But Zachary's daily fight for life is the catalyst of many stories of inspiration. We witnessed a young lad take on so many challenges and amazingly rose to each and every one. We learned a lot about the human spirit through Zachary's plight and through it all he gave us much more than he received.

Deanna and I are certainly bound to hold our breaths a little when Zachary takes on the role of an active child. Whether he climbs a tree or falls off of a bike we will always have the new organs in mind. It will take some time for this adjustment – both for this child and his parents.

Due to his young age, Zachary is very unlikely to remember any part of this life. For that we are grateful. In the future when he gets older, Deanna and I will share with him our memories of this experience. We will tell about his ability to face adversity and overcome incredible odds. We will tell him how his strength inspired a multitude of people. Hopefully he will listen in awe but I suspect that he will only want to borrow the car keys and drive to the mall.

No matter what his reaction may be, the simple fact is that a small child entered the world with the odds stacked against him and yet battled his way back to health. It is not clear just how he did it, yet he did and thousands of people witnessed his progress.

Today is the first day that we step out into the world away from the hospital walls. We now have our family back and are ready to resume a normal life.

But what is normal in this day and age?

Epilogue, by Deanna Johnson

Looking back I had a difficult time deciding on a college major. At first, I chose Hospitality Management, but soon realized that I would need to work many evenings, holidays, and weekends. I decided that route was not for me. I then discovered that I wanted a career in which I could help people and thus finally decided on Human Resources. I graduated with a Bachelor of Science in this field and worked in many areas of industry including automotive and healthcare. This last industry sparked my interest in physical therapy and I decided once again to change my major and pursue a Masters Degree in this field. I finally felt that I had chosen the right career specializing in Pediatric Physical Therapy.

Who knew that this decision would be the best choice to help my own child? I have been working as a Pediatric Physical Therapist for the last 7 years and never thought I would be using my skills to help my own son.

I remember a poem titled "Welcome to Holland" written by Emily Perl Kingsley. This short story inspired me as a new physical therapist and continues to guide me now as a parent with a child with special needs. Zachary has a long road to recovery ahead of him. In addition to intense physical therapy, he also needs occupational therapy, speech therapy, hearing and feeding programs. Yes, the journey will be slow, but what a ride it will be.

It is nice to finally have our family all together under one roof since the past two years have been such an emotional roller coaster. But our worries do not end here, for we will need to monitor him for signs of rejection of his transplanted organs for the rest of his life. Additionally, we will probably need to learn a new language... that is Sign Language. Our hopes of having the boys together in the same classroom at school or listening to them talking late at night appear to be gone.

Many people ask me, "How do you do it?" and comment that "we are so strong". But you do what you need to do for your child simply because you love them. I truly hope that this book makes people laugh, cry, and helps them to understand of our life caring for a medically fragile child. I am so proud of my son. He is such a fighter. I hope and pray that he will lead a healthy and happy life as he grows old with his twin brother, Aidan, and baby sister, Madeline.

I feel blessed to have brought Zachary into this world for I know he is destined for great things. He has inspired and reached so many. Don't be surprised if there is another book on the horizon. Zac is just beginning his life now... a life outside of the hospital and away from Bed 15.

I hope the view is much nicer.

Acknowledgements ◇

To my wife Deanna, your elegance and grace under the pressures
of the unknown were truly above and beyond all expectations. You
rose to each and every occasion without falter or hesitation and in
doing so set the bar of parenthood that much higher. ◇

Grandparents: Dick & Joyce Johnson ◇ Chris & Bob Joss ◇

Fundraising Volunteers: Kate Garmey ◇ Debbie Gill ◇ Christine
Riganati ◇ Josh Wolf ◇ and by association: Brian Garmey ◇ Matt
Gill ◇ John Riganati ◇ Denise Wolf ◇

Proofreaders: Ginny Korecko ◇ Chris Joss ◇ Joyce Johnson ◇ Traci
Thorpe ◇ Laura Dreves Dabolish ◇

Friends & Family: Jane & Ralph Munoz ◇ Dora Milliner ◇ Tom &
Michelle Joss ◇ Jerald & Misty Pruner ◇ Nikki Jaskiewicz ◇ Jill Heinz
◇ Kim & Corey Moore ◇ Wayne and Jodee Reid ◇ Dr. Nicole
Chandler ◇ Staff at Highland Plaza ◇ Staff at The Ronald McDonald
House (Shadyside, PA) ◇ Annapolis Mothers of Multiples ◇ Greater
Severna Park Mom's Club ◇ Mike & Julie Moundalexis ◇ Larry &
Caroline Smith ◇ Tom & Jeannie Bennett ◇ All of the wonderful
neighbors who provided assistance with our various fundraisers ◇

All the doctors, nurses and therapists at the following: The
University of Maryland Medical Center ◇ The Johns-Hopkins Medical
Center ◇ Children's Hospital of Pittsburgh ◇ The Children's Home ◇

All of the generous people who contributed to Zachary's fund ◇

Special thanks to the transplant surgeons and staff at Children's
Hospital of Pittsburgh: Dr. George Mazariegos, Dr. Rakesh Sindhi,
Dr. Kyle Soltys, Dr. Geoffrey Bond ◇ Patti Harris ◇

Printed in the United States
131638LV00003B/1-24/P